NOT WHO I ONCE WAS

MY UNUSUAL PATH TO BECOMING A SURGEON

DR. JAMES E. HARRIS JR., MD

NOT WHO I ONCE WAS

For information, contact:

James Harris Jr, MD, FACS

jamesharrisjrmd@gmail.com

www.jamesharrisjrmd.com

Instagram: jamesharrisjrmd

Table of Contents

Preface

It has taken many years for me to accept that there is no "right time" to write my story, one not always filled with happiness. I began this process over a decade ago, thinking I had accumulated enough unique tragedies during my journey to becoming a surgeon. Expelling the words sometimes feels like coughing up shards of glass, but as time passes, the edges become less sharp, and the smaller fragments become indistinguishable from sand. Time does not heal all wounds; some fester if not treated correctly, often leaving the worst scars. My hope is that sharing my story may help others learn how to heal and live with the scars of their own.

Learning to move on while paying emotional respect to past traumas can be challenging. Moving forward in the middle of a storm can be dangerous, but so can remaining still. Riding out the storm and waiting for the sun to rise works for most of us, but some circumstances may never change. What then for those whose state of change is beyond repair? Some will simply wait, hoping and praying for a miracle that may never arrive.

This can lead to despair. During my lowest times, I have found myself drawn closer to God. In the book of Matthew, Jesus states that it is easier for a camel to pass through the eye of a needle than for a rich person to enter the kingdom of God. I believe our worldly possessions can, in fact, lead us further away from God. The miracle for me has been realizing that despite my accomplishments and possessions, it is the most devastating tragedies that have pulled me closer to the Lord. For those who are suffering, I suggest accepting the day's circumstances, looking to God for strength, and finding happiness in what is present or within reach.

As a surgeon, I have been inspired countless times by patients who, despite losing certain functions due to severe health conditions, have found ways to adapt and make progress. As the parent of a disabled son, I am inspired by my child's joy in listening to music and his pride after hitting a series of correct notes on the keyboard using his one functional hand. Once a track-and-field star on his way to college, he became severely disabled after a traumatic brain injury. I like to think of myself as strong-willed and dedicated, but suffering such devastation and still finding happiness is, I believe, the highest level of accomplishment. Human accomplishments certainly have limitations, but we shine and inspire others through what we can do despite our limits. In this memoir, I hope to share many of the challenges I have encountered and how I either overcame them or learned to adapt and ultimately find happiness.

CHAPTER 1

The Crack Years

When I dream or have nightmares, I still find myself back in my childhood home. Our house was the one about halfway down the street, with a big mulberry tree in the front yard. I am forever trapped within its cracked and dingy white walls, which were filled with roach eggs. The crawl space was shared with rats and roaches. Berries from the tree were carelessly tracked in by those who frequented our home, leaving stains in the 70s-era shag carpet that, over time, looked as though they were part of the pattern. In my room, with the door closed, I was never afraid. I had driven a nail halfway through the doorframe, which was then bent into the shape of an "L." I could twist the nail from side to side as a way of locking it. I thought I was a genius when I came up with that. It kept out the crazy people who frequented and even lived in my home. Most of the crazy people were family members. The only one who was sane, in my young eyes, was Mama—my grandmother who raised me.

The eyes of a crackhead were always a bit off. For strangers who came to the door asking for my dad or my uncle, you could always see the brief look of desperation because they were fiending for a fix. Their eyes were not shy, and they automatically scanned all around the house as they came in, pausing briefly on things of potential value. As these people passed by me, their sour smell was somehow still present, even while I held my breath. They seemed unaware that I watched them. I knew better than to leave any of my toys lying around because things had a way of going missing when we had company.

My room was right next to the bathroom where they would smoke crack. When I was between the ages of seven and thirteen, my father, my uncle, one of my aunts, and multiple "family friends" used that bathroom as their sanctuary. Crack has a musky, sweet odor, one that could probably be mistaken for incense by a layperson; I was able to identify this smell by the time I was nine. The back wall of the closet in my room created a thin, narrow barrier to the bathroom on the other side. Nails had once been hammered through this wall to hold up various pictures over the years. After the pictures came down and the nails came out, the holes remained. Through these holes, I was able to watch them.

The glass crack pipe was the popular choice for smoking, but some would fall back on various other contraptions, I assume, because they had lost their pipe while on a delusional rampage. Considering the depth of their drug-induced insanity at times, the ingenuity always surprised me. It was like watching that old television show *MacGyver*: an old soda can, a toilet paper roll with some tin foil; you name it, give them the resources and they would make it into a crack pipe. Desperation is an understatement when it comes to describing people who are hooked on crack. Some of their makeshift pipes would get so hot that they burned their lips. It was so strange to watch it happen. They would react to the pain when the scorching-hot pipe touched their lips, but then go straight back to it for another hit. Once they got that rock, it was going to get smoked.

When I first discovered the peepholes, I was afraid they would see me. I did not fully understand what I was watching. Sometimes I would shift to a different peephole to get a better view, and the floorboard would creak or the box I was balancing one foot on would shift. Their heads would turn, and I would quickly avert my gaze and move back. They were so focused on their goal of smoking that little white rock that the sound was not enough to distract them to the point of investigating.

Some acted stranger than others when they smoked crack. Most tried to appear normal in an attempt to keep Mama from knowing what they were doing. Mama and my Aunt Pat were the only ones who did not use. But my father was by far the worst. At baseline, my father was already paranoid, but when he was using, you knew it. More than three hundred pounds, he'd pace the floor, drenched in sweat, opening and closing doors, locking and unlocking windows. Even when I was in my room with the door closed, I could tell what was going on by the frantic sounds of his footsteps throughout the house. On several occasions, the weight of each step reverberated through the baseboards enough to wake me from sleep. I remember feeling afraid that there was an intruder or that we were being raided by the police. On multiple occasions, I tried to keep him from going outside when he was high. I wanted to protect myself from the embarrassment of the neighborhood kids seeing him in his "cracked-out" state. One time, when I was around nine years old, I thought I could use all my strength to keep that three-hundred-pound man in the house by force. I was mistaken.

I grabbed his arm by the elbow when he reached for the front door. I was met with a quick glance through eyes that did not seem to recognize who I was. It was not my dad, but a monster who somehow stole my voice, like in one of my nightmares where I was unable to scream. My mouth opened, but the sound remained trapped in my lungs, making my chest feel as though it was about to explode. I was thrown on the couch, unable even to exhale. My muscles involuntarily tightened as I curled into a ball, preparing to be hit. My father had never struck me, but everything in that moment suggested that the man with the empty, unrecognizing eyes was not my father. The crack was like rabies to his mind. I was facing Stephen King's *Cujo* in the form of a man.

Instead of feeling the impact of a fist, I felt his hands moving down to my waist. He started to push his huge hand into my pockets. His fingers felt like multiple little mice had entered my pocket and were searching for some other way to escape. I did not initially understand what was happening, but my fear immediately transformed into anger, which broke my paralysis. My

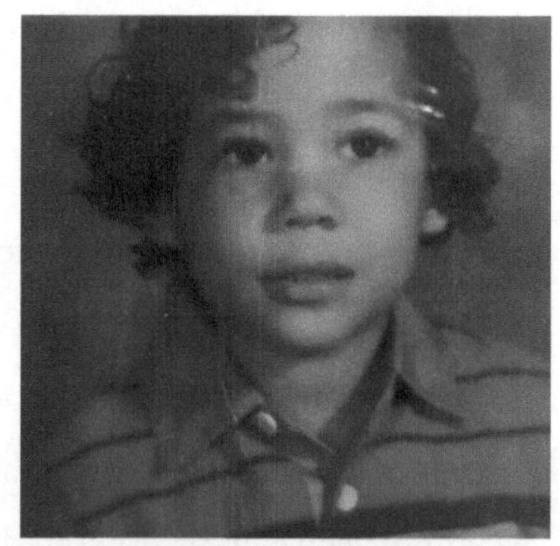

CHILDHOOD PHOTO OF ME AROUND THE TIME CRACK TOOK OVER MY HOME

scream finally escaped as a young boy's shrill, which probably could not be distinguished from that of a girl. He was not fazed. He pulled my front pockets inside out. His focus then shifted as his eyes showed a feeling of hope. He picked at a white ball of lint in my pocket and closely inspected it. He held me down with one hand while the other raised the potential crack rock toward the light from the window in his field of view.

As I screamed helplessly on the couch, Mama came from behind him, swinging a frying pan and yelling at him to get out. I think she may have struck him at least once because he quickly retreated out the front door in the way an injured bear, shot by a hunter, would scurry off into the woods. A couple of years passed before I saw him again.

CHAPTER 2

Never Trust a Crackhead

Around the time I was in second grade, most of my family, except for Mama and my Aunt Pat, were getting high on crack. That smell would seep into my room when they smoked in the bathroom. Unlike the magnetic effect that the aroma of freshly baked cookies has, crack repelled me, making me want to get away. One Saturday morning, while watching cartoons in my room, that smell percolated into my little safe haven. I became quite annoyed as to which crackhead family member of mine was disrupting my peace this time. My father's presence was the most obvious because of his heavy steps and wild antics, but for the others, I'd leave my room to investigate. When I poked my head through my door, I noticed my uncle's girlfriend, Lisa, also a crackhead, was about to head out the front door, so that left my uncle as the likely suspect for disrupting my Saturday morning cartoons with his repulsive smoke. Looking for a reason to get away, I asked Lisa where she was going. She said she was walking to the little neighborhood store a few blocks away to get groceries.

Usually, I wouldn't go anywhere with Lisa because she was often under the influence of something, but she did not look high this time. Besides Lisa's drug problem, she also had a dark history that scared me as a child. She was at one time married to an older man who was retired and received various monthly checks while he was alive. Lisa had her drug problem during his later years and often used much of his income for her addiction. Her husband passed away, reportedly of natural causes, but rather than reporting his death immediately, she kept his body in the bedroom of their home for a few months after his death to continue collecting his checks. I was never told whether she faced any charges or served any time for this, but regardless, I always thought of her husband's body rotting away and turning into a mummy while she remained in the house. That memory gave me pause about asking to go with Lisa, but that musky, sweet smell was getting pretty bad, and I thought I might be able to get some candy if I tagged along. It was pretty rare for any of my crackhead family members to get me any of the good stuff, but back then there were nickel-and-dime candies that I could always convince them to buy for me.

It was a beautiful Saturday morning as we walked out the door. Birds were chirping, the mulberry tree out front was starting to bear fruit, and there was not a cloud in the sky. Plans for going out later with the neighbor kids to play football were high on my list. I yelled out to Mama that I was going to the store with Lisa and grabbed my skateboard. Mama ran that house, but she let me do as I wished most of the time.

The store was only a few blocks away, and there was only one busy street to cross. I rode my skateboard part of the way, going back and forth along the side of the street alongside Lisa. I did not wear a helmet, and I do not recall ever seeing any other kids wearing them back then. I didn't think it was uncool; it just wasn't common back then. If only I knew what was about to happen to me; if only I knew how this knowledge would haunt me more than twenty-five years later with my own son.

A small church across the street from the corner store had a steep ramp that was great to ride my bike down when there were no services going on. I contemplated trying it with my skateboard. If I fell and looked stupid, it was just my uncle's crackhead girlfriend there to make fun of me. As we approached, I saw that there were people standing outside so I had to skip out on the whole ramp adventure. We crossed the street and entered the shop, where I headed straight for the candy aisle. I don't remember what I got or how much; such details likely would have been forgotten anyway, despite what was about to happen. I do remember the exact layout of the store and the family who owned and operated it. My Aunt Pat had a "credit" account with them where she would pay off her bill monthly after each disability check came in. Pat even had a "credit" account at the Popeyes chicken restaurant a few blocks away from the house. The candy aisle was within view of the checkout line. This probably helped dissuade kids from stealing. These folks knew my family, so I never even thought about stealing from them. On the candy aisle, they had all the good stuff around eye level for a kid. Sometimes you could catch a sale where they would sell four for a dollar. Usually, it was the less popular brands like Whatchamacallit or Rolos, but to me, candy was candy; it was all good. The bottom of the aisle had all the bite-size nickel-and-dime candies. I grabbed a few of my favorite choices and put them in the basket. We checked out and began walking back home, across the one semi-busy main street.

I was a few steps behind her and didn't look for oncoming traffic. I suppose I thought it was safe being close enough to her, but I was wrong. *Sesame Street* taught me to look both ways and to cross the street with an adult, but it never taught me to mistrust an adult who happens to be a crackhead. I missed seeing the car approaching on my left side. Lisa was several steps ahead of me and out of the line of impact. I was not so lucky. According to witnesses, when the car hit me, my head and body struck the windshield, breaking it, and I was thrown more than thirty feet as the driver slammed on the brakes. I have scattered memories surrounding this event, but the most prominent is of waking up on the asphalt and seeing blood and glass all over the street around me. I couldn't move and was terrified. I don't remember anyone being around me at first, but after losing consciousness and then waking again, my father had magically appeared and was pacing back and forth, freaking out. He was frantic and crying, saying over and over that I was going to be okay. I lost consciousness again and then woke up briefly as I was being loaded into the ambulance. My final memory of that day was waking up with my leg placed in a cast and being cleaned up by a nurse who was wiping my face and combing pieces of glass out of my hair. This was back in the day when Jheri curls were the style, so I had a bunch of grease in my hair. I remember how the glass stuck to the comb with globs of the hair grease. I often joke that the hair grease absorbed the impact on my head and saved me that day, but I would be lying if I did not acknowledge that this was the first miracle of my life. The amount of force it takes to break a windshield is not small, and the distance my body was thrown would suggest an extremely high likelihood of injury to major organs. Most commonly, such trauma leads to death from a major brain injury or other serious injuries that would require emergency surgery; I only had a broken leg.

While my lack of memories surrounding the accident is likely due to a concussion, the absence of other injuries is hard to reconcile in my scientific mind. Those who believe in God often pray for miracles, but we often overlook the miracles that happen to us. Until writing this, I had never before considered what happened to me as a miracle. To be struck by a car, have my head and body break the windshield, and then be thrown more than thirty feet away from the vehicle without any other injuries— besides the femur fracture and some abrasions—is hard to believe. When I think of accidents in which cars strike a deer at high enough speed for it to hit the windshield, I would bet that the poor deer ends up as roadkill. If I didn't have the femur fracture, one could argue that perhaps I wasn't hit that hard, but to break the femur and the windshield cannot be overlooked. Without hesitation, I give credit to God in saying it was a miracle.

I was unable to walk without crutches for several weeks after the accident. One day, I answered the phone at the same time my grandmother did and eavesdropped on a conversation between her and my doctor. I was a nosy little kid. He was telling her that I needed to increase my mobility and start bearing weight on my leg if I wanted to walk normally again. It had been several weeks during which I was barely moving around with my crutches. I had been doing very little weight bearing out of fear of causing further injury to myself, but after hearing that I could be setting myself back by not moving around, I started walking on that leg immediately. My leg was stiff and out of condition. It hurt like crazy to put weight on it. This was the first time I started to realize how much power my mind had over my body. Before picking up that phone and hearing the doctor say that I could walk, I was disabled. Moments later, after hearing the doctor say it was okay for me to bear weight before they cut the cast off, I was up and

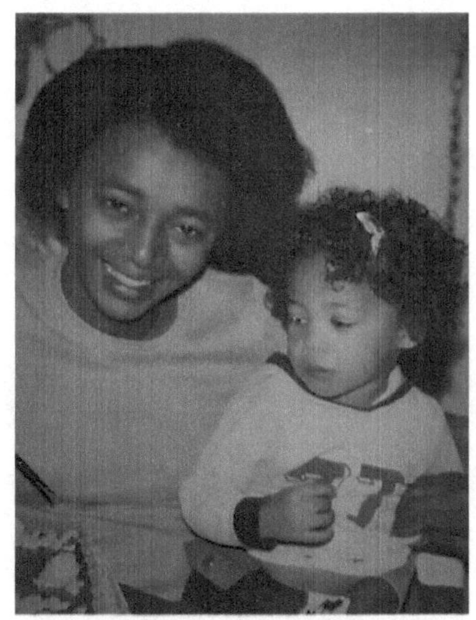

ME WITH MY AUNT PEARL JUST BEFORE THE CRACK YEARS

moving around. I walked so much that the cast started to crack at the bend of the knee by the end of the week. Similar to the title character in *Forrest Gump*, who started running to the point that his leg braces shattered and fell off, I was moving around so much that I could fully bend my hip and knee before the cast was removed. After its removal, I returned to school walking and running normally. The awareness that *it had been my own mind that held me back* led me to realize the potential I possessed to overcome other challenges in life. The fear of getting hurt or of failure is enough to discourage most people from ever pushing to their potential. Many people live their lives always taking the path of least resistance. It is the reason many never chase after their dreams. It requires some level of sacrifice. This tragic event may have led to a bad injury, but I believe it was God's plan to teach me about resilience.

CHAPTER 3

The Lady in the Picture

The photo was somehow seared in my mind. For many years in my early childhood, I recall looking at a snapshot in an old album of my baby pictures, a photo of me as an infant. In it, I'm being held by Mama at one of my Aunt Pearl's basketball games. Aunt Pat (Pearl's older schizophrenic sister who helped raise me) is sitting on Mama's left side, and a white woman is seated on her right. On a number of occasions, I asked Mama and other family members who that lady in the picture was. The bleachers were not that packed, and she seemed too close and too familiar with Mama to be a stranger. The reply was always, "I don't know," or "Just some lady at the game."

One day, after my father had returned sober after one of his absences, he beckoned me to my room to sit beside him on the edge of my bed. I was still in grade school at the time, around 10 years old.

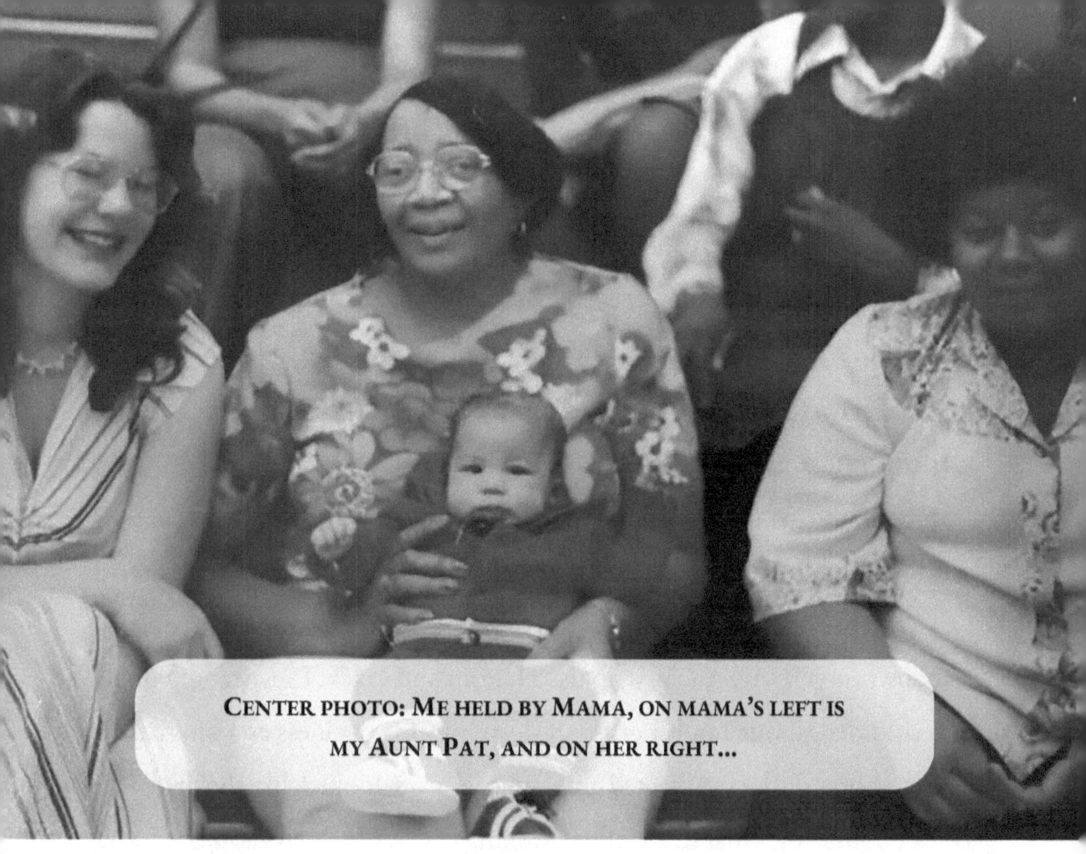

I had just returned from playing outside with the neighbor kids and found my father holding the photo album in his lap, with the page open to that photograph of me and Mama with the white lady in the picture. I had a deep ache in my gut and felt that something was wrong. I did not ask him who that was, as I usually did. My father asked me, "Do you know who this is?" I shook my head no, but felt inside that the truth of what had been hidden from me for years was about to be told. He pointed to that white woman in the picture and said, "This is your Mama." Wrong choice of words. Mama was in her room across the hall, unaware that my father was telling me this. Maybe if he had said, "This is your biological mother," it would not have been such an insult and shock, but to replace the woman who raised me with this stranger was too much. Rage and sadness overwhelmed me. I don't remember what I said, but I threw a fit, kicked my giant of a father out of my room, and locked myself in there for hours. The whole house knew what had happened, and my father was told not to come around for a few days while I adjusted to my new reality: my mother was not Mama.

Shortly after the revelation about my birth mother, there was another difficult interaction with a crackhead who was not part of my family. I'd learned not to get involved in the business of crackheads after that situation with my dad, but I didn't think that David was all that dangerous. David was a former boyfriend of my Aunt Pat. He, like others, came to my home to hang out with my uncle, who used heroin and crack. I suspect my uncle also sold drugs, but I never got that deep into his business as a kid. David was a short, dark-complected guy who always looked like he had just finished running a marathon after smoking crack. He always appeared a bit unkempt in his plain white T-shirt with yellow sweat stains under his arms and dirty jeans. He often came to the door making light jokes when I would answer it. His humor made me feel comfortable enough to one day poke fun back at him. That didn't work out so well.

That day, I watched David leaving my uncle's room with beads of sweat running down his face and said something that seemed funny at the time. I can't remember exactly, but it wasn't anything much worse than what he had said to me in the past. He snapped. He sprinted across the room toward me before I had any time to react and grabbed me by my shoulders. I was shaken with such force that I felt as though my neck was going to break. He threw me onto the couch and pointed his finger at me, saying, "Don't you ever mess with me again. Do you understand?!" I remained sprawled out on the couch, paralyzed with fear. "Do you understand?!" A slight nod of my head, my eyes diverted to Mama's door, must have sufficed, because he ran out the door before Mama even knew what had happened. Although David was high, he must have recognized that he had screwed up because he never returned.

After that second incident of being attacked by a crackhead, I chose not to be a victim any longer. I remained isolated in my room most of the time and started lifting weights. I was going through a growth spurt that accompanied many of the other changes of puberty. I thought that if I could become strong, then maybe the next time I could fight back. Anger and hate started to grow inside of me. That feeling of helplessness made me feel disgusted with myself. My innocence and gentle childhood nature darkened. Many hours were spent fantasizing about my revenge. If I could not overpower him (or my next attacker), I had a backup plan. I carried a cheap knockoff of a Swiss Army knife, but I never felt comfortable with the idea of stabbing someone. However, my combination lock fit very well in my hand and made a great sneaky weapon. If held the right way, I could deliver a roundhouse blow to the side of his head. If that failed and he grabbed me, I would either scratch at his eyes or bite him. I spent many hours strategizing about what I would say when I saw him to make him react in the same way he did when he attacked me, but this time I would be ready. I wished he would come back.

A next time never happened for David. He, like many others who are addicted to crack and heroin, died of an overdose on the streets sometime after our last encounter. But my hate and anger lived on after his death, transferable to anyone who might cross me in the future.

The following summer, I entered fifth grade. I started getting into fights, and my grades began to slip. I rarely smiled when not with friends, and if provoked, I would never turn the other cheek. I managed to keep my grades just good enough to stay in the district throughout middle school, but near the end of eighth grade, I was out of control. Besides poor academic performance, I started getting into more trouble and hanging out with the wrong crowd. I separated myself from the privileged kids who once bullied me and started to associate with those who I felt were like me. My girlfriend relationships in middle school were often short-lived, as would be expected for childhood love, but they too were with girls who I felt were, like me, afflicted by darkness. They had been hurt by others, and they were not afraid of my way of being; if anything, they may have been attracted to me because they thought they could fix me.

Many of the kids I went to school with on the "good side of town" had financially well-off families. Some of them spoke of the college funds that their parents had saved up for them and the expensive trips they had taken across the country with their older siblings to visit colleges. My grandmother barely had enough money for us to survive on, let alone to pay for college. We survived on government assistance through welfare, food stamps, and disability checks. I felt out of place in the more affluent school because I was poor. My outlook on education around that time became quite bleak. Although I had aspirations of becoming a doctor as far back as second grade, I felt as though my efforts were futile and lost interest in my education as I approached high school. After I allowed my grades to drop, I was not allowed to continue my education in the same district, so I ended up returning to my side of town for high school, where things only got worse.

Going to school in an area with poverty, gangs, drugs, and very few resources at times felt like going to prison. There were guards and fences in place to ensure no student escaped during the school day. Those who dared to leave without permission before school was out had to plan their escape carefully so as not to be chased down and detained. While school was in session, we *were* prisoners. Most students who would eventually go on to become law-abiding citizens followed the rules and went to class as they were expected so that they could graduate on time. Such students had some sense of direction and understood the importance of getting an education. Perhaps they saw the opportunity in getting their education, or they were just afraid of the consequences of not doing what they were expected to do. I did not see things that way. I lived only for the moment and not the future. I entered a lifestyle of fighting, stealing, and complete disregard for anyone who was not in line with my path.

It is not clear to me whether it was the emotional loss that I felt when I discovered that the lady in the picture was my mother or the physical loss of control that I experienced when my father and David attacked me that played the larger part in my spiritual decline. Mama and my father introduced me to the Bible early in my childhood. I believed in God but never really recognized His presence in my life. In Matthew 19:14 of the Bible, Jesus refers to children and says, "The kingdom of heaven belongs to such as these." It was around this time in my life that I felt I had lost this inheritance.

CHAPTER 4

Worth Killing For?

A full moon illuminated the clear, cool night. I felt exposed. This was not the best way to go unseen with what we planned. The .380 pistol was about the size of my hand. It felt warm as I pulled it out of my pocket and held it low in the passenger-side seat, preparing to pull the trigger. My cousin drove slowly around the corner and glared at me before approaching the house. My eyes were wide, lips tight, taking in every detail. Beads of dew had already started to form on the unkempt lawn of the corner house where we slowed to a stop. I released the magazine to check that it was still loaded for the third time.

Had I already put one in the chamber? I had. That was why I had the safety on, so that I wouldn't make the same mistake twice. A couple of days before, I was in my room with the door locked, practicing how to load and unload the gun. I was only thirteen years old and had borrowed the gun from "Big E" more than a week before. Big E was around 17 years old, making him our oldest friend. He was considered the "OG" and the go-to guy for advice and for weed. But on that day, I had run to his house in desperation when my father tried to run me over with his car. I had never cried in front of any friend before that day. I told Big E everything, as if he were the Godfather.

My dad had a brief relapse with crack that led to a huge fight. He rolled up to his house erratically, as though he were being chased. I was waiting for him just outside his chain-link fence. We had plans that day, but I can't remember what they were. As he pulled up and came to a stop, a cloud of dust rose. I looked at his eyes and saw fear. I looked down the street to see if there was somebody after him. The rest of the block was quiet and barren. The door flew open, and his face was contorted as though he wanted to say something but could not. It was the typical crack face for my dad: a cross between confusion, frustration, and insanity. It was like he was unsure who he was or what he was supposed to be doing. I was shocked to see him like that. It had been years since he had left to apparently get clean. I was still shorter than my dad and less than half his weight, but I rushed at him. He was no longer an immovable force. I pushed him back into the side of the car and began to yell, "What are you doing?" He was unusually soft at initial impact but quite massive, with a dense weight, so he was probably only shoved a foot or two backward into the car.

Though he could have done anything in his state of mind, I didn't believe he could hurt me. Something immediately changed in his eyes, which made me step back. He got in the car and slammed the door. I jumped in front of the car to stop him from driving while high. I had lost all trust in my dad's ability to be rational, so I kept myself a few feet away from the front bumper and off to the side. Before I had a chance to say anything, he accelerated. The same man who panicked after seeing me lying unconscious on the street as a young child, with blood and glass around my seemingly lifeless body, was prepared to drive his car into me. Like a matador, I spun backward off my right foot and into the chain-link fence just a few feet away. The old, junkyard-quality car sped right through where I had been standing. I looked through the cloud of dust. Those dark, blank eyes never looked back in the rearview mirror.

Big E listened as I pleaded my case to borrow one of his guns for protection. If my dad were to return, I would be ready. He reluctantly let me use his .380 pistol but told me not to do anything that I would later regret. I agreed to appease him, but my intentions were not good. I was angry and still in the heat of that fury, which I hid from Big E. Thankfully, time can lead to the dissipation of even the most intense rage. Distracted by thoughts of what would happen if I had to pull the gun on my father the next time he threatened me, and because of my ignorance about how the gun worked, my finger must have pulled the trigger as I cocked it, and the gun went off. The loud bang was like a bomb exploding in my room. "What was that?" my grandmother screamed. "Just a firecracker outside," I said, with only a brief hesitation. "It's the neighbor kids messing around." I don't know if she believed me, but there was no further discussion after that.

I maintained an obsessive-compulsive (OCD) level of caution thereafter. I would click the safety in place, then press it again even harder to make sure it wasn't partly disengaged, three times for good luck, to be certain. Despite these safety checks, I still checked every so often while I kept the gun in my pocket, just in case the safety got clicked off while moving around. It wasn't that easy to do, and it never did, but I would still check anyway. There weren't many opportunities to practice shooting without fear of somebody seeing me, so I had no idea whether my aim was good enough to hit my target. I was pretty good at shooter games like *Duck Hunt*, but not the best; my cousin often beat me. Besides my questionable aim, questions started to fill my mind: *What is my target? Do I just aim for the window of the guy's room? I don't even know which room is his. If he happens to be outside, can I shoot him? What if he has his gun? Do I shoot multiple times? Does he have a younger sibling I could hit by mistake? What about his parents? That saying, "A bullet has no name," couldn't be truer. I was going to shoot up the house without a clear target.*

My cousin was willing to be the shooter, but I needed to have control over what was going to happen. I looked over to see if he looked concerned and I saw emptiness. I tried to mirror the lack of emotion so that I could go through with it. My cousin and I were close growing up. He would visit during school breaks and stay for several weeks at a time. We were often out running the streets, looking for opportunities to make money. There were no discussions of honest earnings, like mowing lawns or getting a summer job at the neighborhood store. We were two idiots scheming to make fast cash. Although we devised big plans, like robbing a bank or one of those armored trucks, none of these schemes ever saw the light of day. Some aspect of each plan always seemed too risky. Most of our crimes were small-scale, low-yield, and pretty stupid.

We did, however, get into a number of conflicts while running the streets, including one with a neighbor from around the block who was about to be our intended target.

Like many bad encounters, this whole scheme started benignly. We were walking to a nearby store to buy some snacks one evening and came across a guy who was drunk and/or high, staggering away from the store. Upon closer inspection, I recognized him as a neighbor from around the block. As we stared, we must have given off a vibe that we were "mean-mugging" him. Mean-mugging is a demeanor adopted in the ghetto, meant to send a message that you are not to be messed with. This goes beyond trying to look tough while minding your business. It goes the extra mile, involving a hateful, intentional glare directed at your intended target. Over time, I learned that mean-mugging was more likely to get you killed than to deter trouble. Most folks would avert their gaze to avoid trouble, but those weren't the problematic ones. The ones who were crazy enough to stare back were the ones to worry about. It was just a matter of time before an encounter would happen.

The intoxicated guy staggered toward us, barely noticing we were there until he caught a glimpse of our stares. He challenged us with his own mean mug, then followed with harsh words. "What the f*** are you looking at?" he asked. We started to argue in response, but then he motioned to the gun he was holding just inside his jacket pocket. He spewed other words of intimidation after seeing we had nothing to say. Our words became lodged deep in our stomachs as they churned. We just stared cautiously; our feet frozen to the pavement. He watched as our initial challenging glare melted into one of despondency. He moved on after having his say without ever having to take the gun out of his pocket, but the damage had already been done; we had been publicly disrespected.

I had the .380 pistol at home, and thankfully I didn't have it on me when we crossed paths with that neighbor. If I had, my ego might have led to a shootout in front of the neighborhood store. Instead, we walked away silently, went home, and plotted for a few days. We initially planned to find the guy later that night, but after the anger and embarrassment had settled, it seemed foolish to look for trouble. My cousin disagreed, but it was my butt on the line if something went wrong. He'd return home after the summer break, while I remained behind, vulnerable. He wanted to make an example of him, but there were several problems with this idea. The most obvious dilemma was that there were witnesses at the store who could identify us as having had a negative interaction with the guy. The cops would have had no trouble figuring out who did it.

A few more days went by before we saw the guy again. We immediately recognized him as we walked past the same store, but he didn't seem to notice us. We thought he probably didn't remember us because he had been so drunk or high. Instead of being thankful for this and moving on, we used this as an opportunity to plan our revenge. Our logic was that if he didn't remember us, then he wouldn't know it was us who shot up his house. This could have been flawed logic. This time, the guy wasn't drunk and might not have had his gun with him. There were two of us, and he was alone. He might have recognized us but, being sober in that moment, had enough sense to act like nothing ever happened. Nonetheless, we began to strategize.

I had never done a drive-by shooting or shot at another human being before. Even though I was still pissed at the guy, I was not prepared to potentially take his life over this. Enough time had passed that my anger and shame from the public disrespect had dissipated. We thought we had a reputation to protect. We were a couple of dumb teenagers who thought we were the center of the universe. What happened did matter to us, and if left unreconciled, there would be future turmoil in our world. His actions against us could not go unchecked.

We waited until after midnight, in the early hours of the next day, to move forward with the plan. After ensuring the gun was loaded, I clicked the safety off and nodded my head toward the guy's house. The whole neighborhood was quiet, with only the sound of crickets. I was on the passenger side with the window open, sitting on the door with my upper body outside the car and out of my cousin's view as he slowly drove toward the house. I made sure the passenger door was locked, then wedged my feet between the seat and the door to prevent falling if my cousin freaked out and slammed on the gas. I faced the guy's house on the opposite side of the street and steadied my aim. I braced myself in anticipation of the car suddenly accelerating and then opened fire.

I had no intention of shooting at the house or anybody in it, but I wanted my cousin to believe we had accomplished our goal and gotten revenge. From his angle, he couldn't see the direction I pointed the gun as I aimed at the sky. As he drove by, I shot into the air a few times as he sped off. I slipped back into the passenger seat and slid halfway down as though expecting a return of fire. My cousin followed suit, crouching down while gripping the steering wheel, tires screeching as the car sped down the street. It was pretty stupid and risky, but thankfully no one was hurt. My cousin believed I shot into the home, and I got to save face.

There is no excuse for the blatant disregard I had for others, but there must be a reason that so many people share a similar path and so many go as far as to murder. Why do some go from cute little kids in elementary school to aspiring thugs at some point in their adolescence? What happened to my childhood innocence? While I take responsibility for all my actions, there must be a reason that this unfortunate transformation happens to so many kids who live in poor neighborhoods. I'm certain that the environment has an impact, but there must be more to it. I was bused away from the ghetto from elementary school through middle school, but the negative transition still happened to me. I was surrounded by well-off, privileged white people, and I still became corrupt. I never felt like I belonged on the good side of town. My neighborhood followed me to school like a puppy. In the beginning, I tried to hide it. After a few years of unsuccessful acclimation, I learned to embrace my differences and wear the 'hood' as a badge of honor. I was that kid who was bused from the hood and was sent back to the hood because he was a bad person. This persona was counterproductive in the classroom. Teachers took little interest in me, nor did I in them. My grades in high school continued to decline, and I was no longer the smart kid, but the troublemaker.

Despite the heavy influence society has on the image some adopt, I believe that one's moral compass can be greatly influenced by love. Regardless of how I looked or acted as a teenager, I had a deeper set of guiding principles that were instilled earlier in my childhood that directed me.

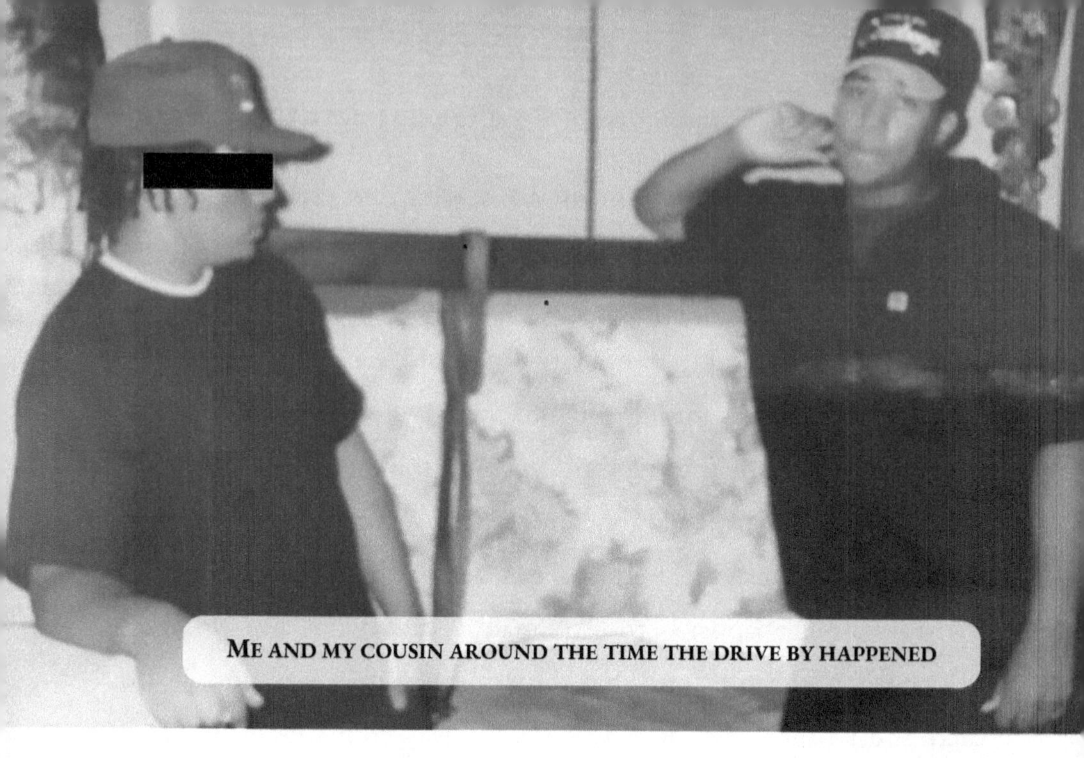

It is never too late to have a positive influence on an individual, but the earlier in childhood it starts, the more likely the child is to shape his or her direction before society does. Social reformer Frederick Douglass said, "It is easier to build strong children than to repair broken men." Perhaps there are critical moments in our childhood where we can be so significantly influenced that it sets us on a path that is difficult to change.

Many opportunities presented themselves in my teenage years where I could have gone too far and seriously hurt or killed someone. That inner voice that was always in the background of my mind took over when I needed it to. I thank God for the love my grandmother gave me early in my childhood. I fear that if I had not been shown love at that critical stage of my development, I very easily could have stepped over the line and ended up on a different path.

CHAPTER 5

One Shot to the Head

The bulldogs that surrounded me have nothing to do with canines. I was raised in southeast Fresno, California, an area largely occupied by a gang called "the Bulldogs," along with multiple smaller gangs. Most of my friends were like me in that they were not fond of the majority of people in these gangs and looked at them as a bunch of followers. By default, we chose to represent the color opposite to theirs. Crips didn't exist in our neighborhood, so we did our own thing. Consequently, this resulted in numerous gang-related fights and shootings, issues still affecting inner cities across America.

It sounds strange, but as teens in the early 90s, my friends and I all enjoyed getting into fights. Gang violence was just starting to get more lethal at the time, so most still fought battles with their fists. We would look for any reason to start an argument; something as small as a dirty look usually sufficed. It wasn't until my friend George was shot that we started to understand how easily a simple fight could evolve into the loss of a life. George was always thought of as the crazy one; he was like Mikey from the old Life Cereal commercial who would eat anything the other kids brought him. George would do almost anything if you dared him to. He was fearless in many ways, which, at the time, I foolishly admired and even aspired to be like. I saw this quality as one of bravery rather than stupidity. Despite some of his crazy antics, he will always be remembered because he would later introduce me to the most important person in my life.

George came over to my house one winter day after getting into an argument with some kid around my age. I was 13 or 14 years old, and George was 16 at the time. They almost got into a fight at the basketball court just down the street after George felt the kid had disrespected him and was determined to fight. The kid somehow convinced George to meet him later that day at a field next to a liquor store in the neighborhood not far from his house. My first logical question to George was, "Why didn't you just fight the kid while you were at the park?"

From George's description of him, the kid was much smaller and would have been an easy fight; he was clearly afraid to fight George at the time and wanted to meet somewhere later to get out of the situation. Given that this guy was smaller than George, my fear was that if he did choose to show up, he would either bring a bunch of guys to jump George or, even worse, bring a gun. I tried to convince George that one of these two things would happen. George replied, "That's why I'm not going alone."

At that time in my life, my definition of what constitutes a true friend was based on a number of things. By far the most important was, "Do you have my back?" If I were in trouble, a true friend would be there to help me through it. Part of what makes a gang feel like a family is this loyalty. This type of love can lead one to murder and death; it is said that the devil can even use scripture for evil, so it is not strange to consider that love can be used as a rationale to justify hatred toward an enemy. Such thinking can create apathy toward those who are not part of the family. I still believe to this day that having your friend's back is key to revealing your dedication, but the way one chooses to help one's friends does not need to warrant dangerous or illegal acts. Unfortunately, instead of doing everything in my power to prevent George from going to meet this guy, I, along with two other friends, went to "back him up."

We all drove to the field next to the liquor store. George sat in the front passenger seat, and I was in the seat directly behind him. Despite my young age, I had been in a fair number of fights before this, and even though this fight wasn't supposed to include me, I felt more anxious than I ever had before. No music was playing in the car, but George seemed to bob his head up and down and slightly side to side as though following a beat. We once talked about what music we'd choose if we were boxers on the way to the ring, and I wondered what song George had in his head.

I had returned the .380 pistol to Big E, so I didn't have a gun at the time. My default weapon whenever I went out without a gun was my perfectly legal combination lock. When held correctly in my hand, it could serve as a dangerous device for blunt trauma to the head. Brass knuckles are illegal in many states, classified as a concealed weapon, but a combination lock can be just as dangerous without the risk of being fined or sent to jail if it were discovered by a cop. Thankfully, I never had to use it because if I did, I very likely could have killed the person I hit.

We arrived at the old, run-down field adjacent to the liquor store, which was in a similar condition. Multiple beer bottles, an old mattress, and various pieces of trash were strewn among the weeds and dirt. An old, broken wooden fence struggled to stand at the back of the field, with an alley behind it.

The store had a couple of burnt-out fluorescent letters on the "liquor" sign. Along with the typical illuminated alcohol advertisements, the paint was falling off parts of the wall that faced the field, and graffiti, spray-painted by members of the local "Bulldog" gang, covered most of the barren parts of the store.

I was happy to see the guy and his friends weren't there yet and started to hope that they wouldn't show. After a few minutes, we heard voices coming from behind the old fence. They started walking through the gap, one at a time. The smallest of the bunch looked up at us as he stepped into the field and began to bark. "Woof! Woof! Woof!" The rest of them followed his lead. "Woof! Wooof! Buuuullll dog! Buuuulll dog!" The Bulldog gang was known for these chants. They'd taken the name of Fresno State University's mascot, the Bulldog. The influence was so widespread that local high schools didn't allow any Fresno State Bulldogs clothing because of the gang affiliation. They were all young, around 13 to 15 years old, and wore big parka jackets. I thought it was funny that they used all that fabric to hide their small frames. Unfortunately, what they were really hiding were their guns.

The main guy pulled his gun and pointed it at George. We had been threatened with guns in the past, and some of us had even been shot at before, but I had never been this close to one, other than my own. I froze, but George walked closer. The kid started taunting George. Without warning, George rushed toward the kid.

Boom!

My heart jumped up into my throat. Was I hit? Before I had time to contemplate my own fate, the answer became clear as I saw George fall face forward.

All I could hear was the ringing of the first thunderous blast, followed by an orchestra of gunshots from the others. I dropped to the ground and crawled to George. He didn't move. I grabbed his shoulder and hip to turn him over and found a single hole in the middle of his forehead, with blood slowly oozing from it. I carefully rested his head on the edge of an old mattress that lay in the field beside him. The shooter and all of his friends fired their guns as they ran; miraculously, neither I nor my other two friends were shot. George didn't move and was completely limp. I took my blue rag out of my back pocket, held it to his head, and looked back to tell one of our two friends to call for help. I found that I was alone. Everyone had run off when the bullets started flying.

I tied the rag to George's head, laid his head back on the mattress, and ran into the liquor store to call for help. The people inside called the police and paramedics while I ran back to George. It appeared as though he was breathing, but in my mind, I thought he was dead. It felt like forever as I waited for the police and ambulance to arrive. All I could do was pray and watch George breathe. Even though I had no regular prayer routine or relationship with God at that time, in desperation, I fell to my knees. I supported his head and stopped the bleeding by holding pressure with my rag over the wound until the paramedics swarmed around me.

Miraculously, George survived. He was in the hospital for more than a week, with most of his time spent in the intensive care unit. We later found out the bullet was from a small-caliber gun and hadn't hit his brain. It had entered his mouth, knocking out a couple of teeth, bounced up through the roof of his mouth, entered his frontal sinus, and exited through his forehead. What I thought was the

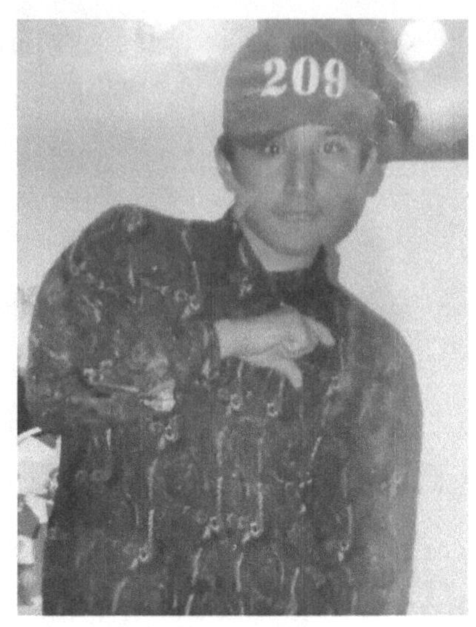

GEORGE BEFORE HE WAS SHOT

point of entry was actually the exit wound. George's lacrimal duct, which allows tears from the eye to drain into the inside of the nose, was damaged on one side in the process, resulting in frequent tearing on that side. The nerves responsible for smell were also injured by the bullet, resulting in an impaired sense of smell, which has recovered significantly over the years.

Despite this close encounter with death, it was still a number of years before George and I completely abandoned our foolish ways. Times have changed since the "good old days" when an argument in the ghetto could be settled with your fists. Now, using a gun has become the new norm in the hood.

George eventually moved on, as I did, and got his life together. He is now working, got married, divorced, and has children. He is one of only a few friends from the past with whom I have stayed in contact all these years. Those who continue living life as a gangster after childhood usually don't make it far. The consequences, or death, catch up with them.

CHAPTER 6

Out of Tragedy Came You

My high school experience was rough because my priorities were misplaced. Much of my focus was on hanging out with friends, girls, and making money. With little concern for my education, I ditched class most of the time, and my grades were horrible. I failed most of my classes and hid this from my grandmother. I even went as far as impersonating her on the phone several times to excuse myself from school. Somehow, the high school administrators believed me, and I repeatedly got away with it. I couldn't maintain this poor performance for long, and after a year of passing very few classes, I fell behind. During my freshman year, I sometimes met up with friends and left before classes even started. Our most common response to concerns about missing too much school was, "F*** school, cuz!" We would yell this at the top of our lungs as we walked off campus like a bunch of cocky idiots, daring the security guards to chase after us. This was part of the fun because some of the guards would give chase. The trick was to leave before the bell rang. If they caught you trying to leave the grounds after the bell rang, the game was on. Only God could have guessed I had an ounce of potential at the time. If those who knew me then were asked to predict my future, most would have guessed I'd become another victim of gang violence or be locked up at some point.

Just before George got shot, he introduced me to his cousin, Rosina. I was only 14 at the time, and she was 16. She was an attractive, older girl I had strong feelings for from the very beginning. We had an awkward first date, with George being the ever-present third wheel. We went to see the Disney movie *Aladdin* at the old Festival Theatre on Blackstone Boulevard in Fresno. I was quite bold on our first date and tried to sneak a kiss during the movie, but Rosina quickly shot me down and ignored me. I kept nudging her to look over at me for a kiss, but she refused to turn her head. I like to think it was because her cousin George was there with us the whole time, but Rosina, now my longtime wife, says I was just too fast and looked like a thug.

Rosina and I had only been on one or two dates when George got shot, but our communication increased significantly thereafter. This tragedy seemed to act as a catalyst, deepening our relationship. Many around us felt we were too close. Rosina's parents thought I was trouble from the very start; I can't blame them for thinking that, because I *was* trouble. Most of my first two years of high school were spent ditching and getting into trouble. I don't know if her parents were aware of the extent of my misbehavior, but it was clear I was not good for her. If a kid were dating my daughter and had done even a fraction of the things I did as a teenager, I would have done everything in my power to talk her out of the relationship.

I fell in love with Rosina quickly. It is strange how love works sometimes. We came from very different backgrounds, with poverty being our only common denominator. Rosina was born in Mexico, the daughter

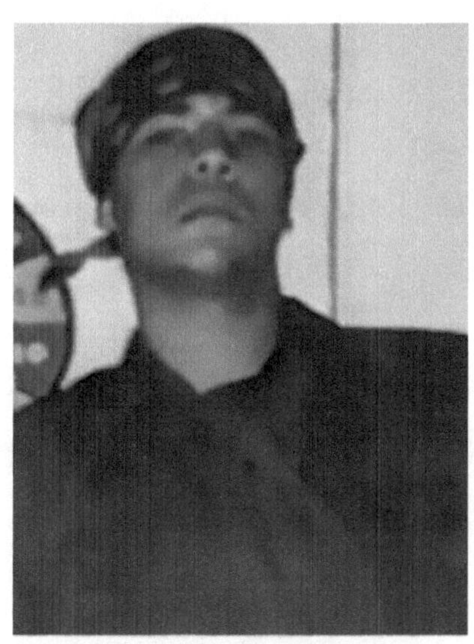

ME AS *THAT* GUY ROSINA'S PARENTS SAW AS TROUBLE (THEY WERE RIGHT)

of migrant farmworkers. She was brought to the United States when she was three years old, crossing a river on her grandfather's shoulders with her mother. She is one of seven children and was raised with a strong sense of duty to her family. From early grade school, she started working in the fields as a child, picking various fruits and vegetables alongside her parents and siblings. She lived with her family on a ranch owned by a farmer who paid them to work the land. To make extra money, her parents would send her and her brothers door-to-door to sell fruits and vegetables. She attended school in the same neighborhoods where she sold produce door-to-door, often feeling embarrassed when she encountered schoolmates while working.

Rosina had, and still has, a beautiful complexion, darker than that of friends who didn't work outside. She was raised in the Catholic

Church and did not wear makeup, unlike some of the other girls. She went to a school where most of the kids were white and was often made fun of for her darker skin. They would call her "Hershey bar." The very thing she was ashamed of—her natural, light chocolate skin, uncovered by makeup—was what attracted me to her at first sight. Her complexion lightened over the years she stopped working outside, though she continued working in the fields throughout part of high school, even after we met. This combination of beauty and fierce work ethic was something I had never seen before. She would make mixtapes for me that introduced me to a love for oldies music. At the time, I only had ears for gangster rap, R&B, and hip-hop, but her thoughtful selection of each song quickly expanded my taste in music. Each mixtape spoke to me, much like the many love letters she wrote to me.

When we first met, I showed little emotion, but Rosina's love penetrated deeply, and I was captivated by her every word and action. I kept every letter from our childhood and memorized every song she selected for each mixtape. To this day, more than 33 years later, I still remember the songs from these mixtapes and even keep some of them on my music playlists.

Externally, I maintained a facade of disinterest, trying to appear tough, but internally, I was all in. We became a couple on January 18, 1993, and on our first Valentine's Day, I bought her a gold promise ring. Every minute we spent together drew us closer and closer. We had no cares beyond this new love, which grew stronger every minute.

Within a few weeks of us becoming a couple, I gave myself my first tattoo on my right arm, using a sewing needle and India ink. I sterilized the needle with a lighter, dipped it in the ink, and scratched the initials R.S.H. into my arm: Rosina Salas Harris.

My early dedication to Rosina negatively impacted my school performance. I frequently skipped classes to spend time with her, failing the majority of them until the middle of 10th grade. Rosina and I grew much closer than her parents would have liked, and she became pregnant before I even turned fifteen. On the verge of dropping out of school and expecting a baby, I found that my high school counselors offered no great advice. To catch up on all my failed classes, I had to leave my regular high school and was sent to Ted C. Wills Restart, an independent-study high school, as a last-ditch effort to avoid dropping out. There, I was allowed to complete all my work at home, dropping off and collecting assignments weekly. With this increased free time, I was able to work full-time at various fast-food jobs and restaurants while simultaneously catching up on my studies.

Although I was determined to turn my life around, it didn't happen overnight. I was far from being an upstanding citizen; I was more like a "menace to society." As a teenager, I harbored goals of success but looked to those around me to define what I valued as achievement. In my neighborhood, those with money and cars were often drug dealers and thieves. I never got involved in selling serious drugs like crack or heroin due to the devastating effects they had created within my family, but I did rob and steal. Many times, I was ashamed of who I was as a teenager and hid my past from others, but remembering who I once was keeps me grounded and thankful for God's grace.

My teenage years were marked by numerous close calls where my foolishness could have gotten myself or others killed. Even before I was old enough to have a driver's license, I was sneaking out and taking family cars for joyrides. This behavior eventually escalated to stealing cars. I learned how to start certain cars without a key, using only a flathead screwdriver to break off the side panel on the steering column and then manipulate the internal mechanism to start the car. My friends and I would look for cars that fit our criteria and pick the nicest one with an open door. Using a "Slim Jim" device to open the door took too much time and often drew too much attention. One of my closest calls, stemming from such poor decisions, involved the last car I would ever take.

I was 15 years old, and Rosina was pregnant with our first son, James—or "Tre" as we called him. She was at her brother's apartment on the other side of town, and I had stolen a Cadillac to visit her. As I approached the apartment complex, I saw her waiting outside. I made an illegal U-turn directly in front of a police officer on the opposite side of the road. Blue lights and a siren went off. Instead of pulling over to be arrested in front of my pregnant girlfriend, I sped off. My adrenaline kicked in, and I suddenly realized how foolish my decision to steal a car had been. Stealing cars had never seemed like a big problem until I faced the reality of getting caught. I stepped on the gas and drove past Rosina. She watched as I sped off, chased by the police, a K-9 unit.

I turned onto the next major street and approached the freeway. I considered turning onto the wrong side of the freeway via an exit ramp, thinking the officer wouldn't follow. However, without my glasses, my blurry vision made that too dangerous. I continued past the freeway entrance and turned down the next major street, which had a moderate amount of traffic. I weaved between cars, gaining some distance. I drove over a wide center divider, crossing to the opposite side of the road. The officer didn't follow directly behind me but took the long way around instead. This gave me enough distance to run a few red lights and turn down a smaller street, taking me closer to home via back roads. Although I was only about 10 minutes away from home, it felt like an hour before I made it to safety. The entire drive, I was terrified the police would appear around every corner. I abandoned the car on the side of the road and walked to my house. For years after that incident, even when I was doing nothing wrong, I panicked every time a police car pulled behind me. I'd mentally review every bad thing I had ever done since kindergarten, worrying that it was finally my time to get caught.

So many things could have gone wrong that day. I could have been caught and charged with grand theft auto and felony evading arrest, and sent to juvenile hall, as some of my friends later were. In my efforts to evade the police, I could have very easily crashed and killed myself or others. For God's sake, in all my panic, I really *had* considered driving onto the wrong side of the freeway as a tactic for escape. My entire life could have gone in a completely different direction that day. That car I stole belonged to someone who worked hard to earn it, and I was using it for a joyride. My decisions showed such disregard for the rights of others that, when I reflect on what I did, it feels like I'm talking about another person. Even though I didn't deserve to get away, I believe God gave me mercy that day. All the possibilities of what could have happened haunted me for some time. The near miss of capture, or even death, helped me reflect on the potential impact on my future and that of my future child.

When I look at what is happening in our disadvantaged neighborhoods, with children subjected to the same external influences that affected me, I see hope because I was once that child. We all have the freedom to make good and bad decisions, but comparing the life of a child raised in poverty to that of one raised in a good neighborhood with a successful, loving family, it doesn't take a genius to predict which child is more likely to become a criminal. It is easy to judge others harshly when one has never walked in their shoes. One's environment does not define them, but it certainly can increase the probability that they will learn from those around them simply due to exposure and ease of access.

I was very fortunate to grow up with a loving grandmother. Many of my friends faced similar challenges—drug-addicted family members, gangs, and poverty—but many lacked that special person, like my grandmother, in their lives. My grandmother was not educated; she never even made it to high school. Still, she always encouraged me and taught me to believe in myself. Throughout my childhood, she spoke highly of me to others, always supportive and proud. Even though I was not her biological child, she raised me as her own. Many of my friends made decisions that led to prison or to failed relationships, often resulting in children with multiple "baby mamas." I can't judge, because I was not far from falling prey to the same outcomes. The only thing that helped me draw the line at critical moments in my life was a strong inner desire to do what was right, instilled in me by my grandmother. I was raised knowing about the Bible, but I didn't truly know God. I believe that God's love can guide us even when we are unaware of it. This love acted like a moral compass, steering me away from wrong decisions at various times in my life. I thank my grandmother, my "Mama," for introducing me to this love at a young age.

Some of my biggest lessons in my teenage years came through close calls. Although a high-speed car chase marked the last time I stole a car, it wasn't the last time I did something that could have landed me in juvenile hall. It's difficult to articulate how I feel about my past, not only because it contrasts with who I am as an adult, but also because it's embarrassing to air my dirty laundry. I haven't omitted these parts of my past from these pages because it wouldn't be fair to act as though I were some perfectly well-behaved kid from the ghetto who followed all the rules and became successful. I hope to reach those who have crossed over to the "dark side." Some have great potential for good and just need to know that change *is* possible. My story is for all, but especially for those who may have made similar mistakes.

CHAPTER 7

If I Could Only Say I Am Sorry

"*Oh no. Oh no.*" My knees started to weaken, and I could barely hold the rotary phone to my ear as Rosina told me, "My mom knows that I'm pregnant. You have to tell your grandma."

I sat down and clutched the phone closer to my ear, afraid that Mama might hear from her room only several steps away. My stomach churned as my heart started to pound in my chest. I stared in the direction of Mama's bedroom door as I cupped my hand over my mouth to whisper, "Are you sure?" It was pretty obvious; that was a dumb question. Rosina was frantic. "Yes!" she said. "I just ran away from my mom as she tried to pull me back by my hair!" Somebody had called Rosina's mom and told her that she was pregnant. Only a few close friends and a cousin knew about Rosina's pregnancy, so we suspected that one of them let the secret slip to one of their parents, who then alerted her mother.

I had been delaying as long as I could, but now my hand was forced. The woman who raised me and held me in high regard was about to have her image of me destroyed. All of the hell that I had been through up to that point was nothing compared to what I had to do. I would have gladly stepped in front of a car again before having to destroy my Mama's image of me. But there was no escaping it; I had to tell her before someone else did. "OK, I'll tell her now," I agreed. I put the phone down carefully, as if I were holding a bomb, and slowly crept back to my room, leaving the door open. "Mama! Can you come here for a minute?" I sat on the side of my bed and looked up at her as she entered my room with a suspicious look on her face. "Mama, sit down. I have to tell you something." I opened my mouth again, but the words did not come out. I started to shake my head from side to side as I stared at the floor. Mama asked, "What's wrong, Buke?" (Buke was an old nickname that all of my family and some friends called me.) Again, I opened my mouth but lacked the courage to tell her. It felt like those words were poison. Keeping them in me, I felt sick. To let them out would hurt her. Shame consumed me. Mama then put me out of my misery and said, "Don't tell me you got that girl pregnant." My eyes widened as the words left her mouth. I still could not get any words out, but instead, I finally shifted my gaze to her eyes and feebly nodded my head to confirm.

"Well, you are just going to have to take care of her."

I have no idea how she guessed, but it didn't matter. Mama's words provided immediate relief, and it was the first time in my life that I experienced such grace. She did not yell at me or tell me that she was disappointed. Mama still loved me, and these few words guided me to the next steps of what I had to do. I was no longer afraid of what the future would bring.

Becoming a father was no longer a fear, but it gave me a new purpose. I had already applied to a few jobs, and not long after, I was hired to work at a fast-food restaurant not far from my house. Rosina came to live with us in that small room where we were going to start our family. We were both too young to move out and didn't have that kind of money to do so. We didn't have to pay for rent or food while staying at home, so my first paycheck went toward buying my son something that I had never had before: a pair of baby Air Jordans. They were not as expensive as the adult size, but it was my way of saying that I would provide for my son the things that I never had.

Before our son was born, Rosina and I both worked full-time to save money and buy all the essentials for having a baby. We turned my small room at Mama's house into a combined nursery even before he was born. Eventually, Rosina made amends with her mom, who accepted her but still did not approve of me. They tried to convince her to leave me and to find an older man who would take care of her, even while she was deep into her pregnancy.

Rosina continued working with her parents in the fields, doing the same kind of work she always had, but she started to have contractions sooner than expected, so her OB/GYN put her on bed rest. This was in complete contrast to Planned Parenthood's original recommendation when she received the positive results of her pregnancy test. They'd given us a card with a number to call for an abortion. Given her young age, aborting the pregnancy was a more logical option from their perspective, but this was never a consideration for us. We felt that our child would be a blessing to our lives and that we would commit to each other and provide a better life for our child than we ever had.

I hustled some, making a little on the side by selling weed, but my main focus was on working and trying to get through high school. While I would like to say I was completely transformed by the new responsibility, I still had the same mindset with regard to doing dirt. My interests were the priority, and I cared very little for those who were outside of my circle. My disregard for others still allowed me to take part in crimes that could have taken away my freedom. My desire for material possessions enslaved me. My ambitions for worldly things nearly led to my demise on many occasions.

The birth of my son did dampen some of the carelessness of my actions. That day was both transformational and terrifying. Seeing Rosina go through the pain of more than ten hours of labor made me feel helpless. I wanted to take the pain from her. I stared at the monitor that showed the contractions starting so I could anticipate the next round of misery, and each time I looked to her as she tried to use the breathing techniques we were taught. She squeezed my hand as the contractions peaked. I willed the pain to go away and watched the contraction monitor decline, her relief showing in a slowing of her breath. When the time came to start pushing, it took several rounds of agony to finally deliver our son. There was immediate relief and celebration in the room as our son cried. We both cried and laughed simultaneously as he was placed in Rosina's arms. I was given the scissors and allowed to cut the umbilical cord. I studied his face and every part of his body, thankful that he was alive and healthy. There was a seed planted at that moment which would later serve as the turning point for my transformation away from the lifestyle I was living, but that transformation took some time.

My last near-miss occurred as we approached our son's first birthday party. I was 16 years old and working around 40 hours a week between two part-time jobs, all while going to an independent-study high school. Rosina was also working, and we were saving up money to move out of my grandmother's house that year, but we didn't have enough funds to have a birthday party for our son. We had planned to take him to Chuck E. Cheese and invite friends and family, but we hadn't realized that between moving and throwing a party, there would be extra expenses. We needed a security deposit and other costs associated with moving into adulthood, so we didn't have the money for this event. The first of the month is when many folks get paid through work and from government assistance, but none of my family had any money to spare, so I devised a plan to get money.

One of my best friends, who lived close to me, had a house across the street from a housing project. The first of the month was a busy time around this area for the drug dealers because of all the government checks cashed by people who lived in the projects. I never got into serious drug sales due to the negative impact crack and heroin had within my family, but I was far from innocent. I didn't make a habit of it, but I did rob and steal on a few occasions when I needed money, and my last time doing so was another one of those close calls where, if I had been caught, it could have ruined my life. More importantly, the trauma and harm I caused the victim is something that cannot be measured but outweighs any other aspect of this story.

My friend's house was not only across the street from the housing projects but also next door to a convenience store that cashed checks. My friend was often involved with many of our plans, but because he was the one with relatively higher morals, he usually distanced himself by serving as the lookout so as to keep his hands clean. If we got caught, he could deny any involvement. My plan was to rob somebody who had just cashed their check at the convenience store. My friend's part was to simply leave his back door open so that I could have a place to hide immediately after the deed was done. I left his house through the back door, which led to an alley behind his house and to the back of the store. I hung out for several minutes as if I were waiting for the bus, and then I found my intended target: a young woman with a thin-strapped purse hanging at her side. A common thief will usually look for easy targets. Houses without alarms that have their lights off are more likely to get broken into. In the same way, most of the cars I had stolen had an open door. It took too much time to jimmy open a lock, and breaking a window was too loud and messy. If the woman had a thick strap hanging across her body, or if she had been with a group of people, I would have passed her by and waited until an easier target came along.

I followed her into the store to confirm that she was, in fact, cashing a check. Carrying large amounts of cash is quite dangerous. Certain celebrities in the music industry flaunt their money by carrying enormous amounts of cash as if they have either zero street smarts or a death wish. Unmarked cash cannot be traced, so you become a huge target if it is known that you carry a considerable amount of money. There are meth addicts who would kill somebody over twenty dollars, desperate for their next fix.

I watched as she walked straight to the counter and handed over her check. I left before the transaction was even completed. I didn't want to draw any attention, so I waited outside by the street. As the woman walked out the door and approached the corner, I snatched the purse from her shoulder and ran into the alley toward my friend's backyard.

I went to open the back door, but it was locked. Extreme panic flooded through my body as I stood there with nowhere else to go. Had I been seen leaving the alley and entering the backyard? For a brief moment, I thought I would take a chance and just run all the way home, but this would have been far too risky since people had been drawn to the woman's scream for help. The first place they'd look would be down the alley where I ran. I stood frozen at the back door for what felt like a few minutes but was probably more like a few seconds, knocking without any response. I didn't know if my friend had fallen asleep or if he got cold feet and didn't want to get involved. I knocked progressively louder without a response. Again, after what felt like a few minutes but was likely just a few seconds, the door was still locked, and I was standing outside, holding a stolen purse.

I made an executive decision and kicked the back door in. The wood around the lock fractured with the first kick. As soon as the back door flew open, I saw my friend's mom standing just beside the kicked-in door. She was quite startled and screamed. She then started yelling, "What did you do, Buke?! What did you do?!" I recall she slapped my arms a few times while yelling at me but the adrenaline was so high that I likely wouldn't have felt it if she had started punching me. I frantically opened the purse, grabbed a handful of food stamps, and gave them to her, saying in a hushed voice, "Please just let me stay here for a little bit." This was my best friend's mom, and she was like a second mother to me, so it was either our history or the food stamps that made her give in. I shoved them into her hand, and that bought me passage into their home. She ushered me into the back room as she angrily muttered expletives under her breath. My friend acted as though he knew nothing about what had happened. I listened from the room as the situation grew more chaotic when his mom noticed the arrival of police cars at the store next door. She became increasingly anxious about harboring me in their home, not knowing if I had been seen.

As time ticked, my friend told me that his mom said I had to go. Police cars were still in the parking lot next door, and they were afraid the police would come over looking for me. I changed my sweater and walked out the back door, feeling certain I was about to be caught. Not only was I leaving while the police were right next door, but my friend's mom made me take the stolen purse with me because she didn't want them to come in and find it on her property. I removed all the money and remaining food stamps from the purse—a few hundred dollars—and shoved the purse under my sweater. I walked out of the alley, opposite the direction of the store, without looking back. Feeling vulnerable was a huge understatement; I felt like I had a neon sign flashing over my head that said, "Criminal here. I did it. Come and get me."

As I approached the end of the alley without anybody flagging me down or yelling at me, I peeked back and saw that the alley was empty, so I quickly dropped the purse between a few trash cans before turning the corner.

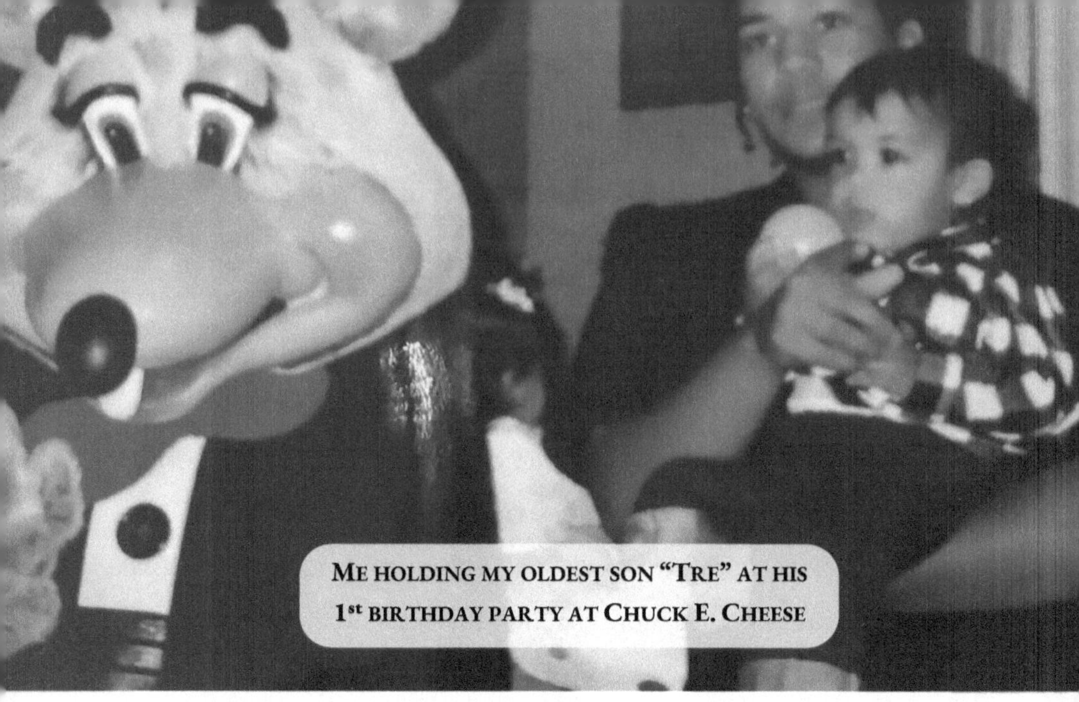

I felt a small amount of relief but still had about half a mile to get home. I stayed on the smaller neighborhood streets and had to pass two major streets to get there. I somehow managed not to see a single police car the entire way. My anxiety was so high that if the police had approached me, I might have panicked and run instead of playing it cool. After getting home, I still played it cool, making a reservation for Chuck E. Cheese. Any guilt was pushed aside by focusing on the future. Bad things in my past were easily pushed to the back of my mind, but they never went away. More than 30 years has passed, and what I did as a teenager still haunts me to this day. I had little concern at the time regarding the impact that my decisions had on the lives of my victims; I only cared about my wants and needs. There is no excuse for such behavior, but as I matured and turned away from such negative acts, I have learned to accept my past and become more understanding of others who have made similar mistakes. I did not deserve it, but God gave me grace when I was at my worst. I am sorry. I am still so sorry.

CHAPTER 8

Words Alone Could Get You Killed in the Ghetto

Hate and anger developed throughout my childhood and festered for many years. These emotions can be dangerous if left unchecked. As a teenager, I saw them as a tool and an asset to be used when I needed them. I also believe that evil thrives in such conditions, and that is when the line of immorality is sometimes crossed. Most of the time, I never came close to crossing that line, but there was one incident that would have ended all that I had if it were not for what I believe was a miracle.

When I was 16, we were living on our own in a poor neighborhood that folks called "Sin City." Often, when I was at work, my wife would go to her mom's house with our son on her days off. I was working at a truck stop as a dishwasher at night and a busboy during the day. One day while I was at work, Rosina called me frantically saying that she had been confronted while walking from her mother's house to the neighborhood store with our son. An older teenage girl who was with a group of boys claiming to be gang members decided to target my wife because of the color of the clothes she was wearing. They were all gathered outside a house across the street from where my wife was walking, and they started yelling profanities about what she was wearing. The teenage girl seemed to be the main one acting tough, and she decided to run across the street and push my wife while yelling at her for walking down their block wearing the colors she had on. Obviously, my wife was scared not only for herself but for our son, who was not even two years old at the time. The girl was in my wife's face, yelling at her and trying to provoke a fight. Rosina explained to them that she had no affiliation with any gang. Eventually, after the girl got her fill of acting like an idiot, they all backed off and allowed my wife to move on with our son.

When Rosina told me this, I immediately left my job and drove home to get my shotgun before meeting up with her. This gun was meant only for home protection, but in this situation, having it with me was the first thing that came to mind. I quickly pulled into our apartment parking lot and jogged to our place, hoping none of the neighbors would be around. I grabbed the gun from under the bed and wrapped it in a thick blanket. I carried it awkwardly, fully aware that if I was seen there would be little doubt as to what it was. I had contemplated sticking the shotgun down my pant leg and then walking stiff-legged out to the parking lot, but this looked even stranger, and I would then have to take the gun out of my pants in plain sight to store it in the car before sitting down. I had used this strategy once before when I went out to the alley behind the complex in the middle of the night to practice shooting it the day after I bought it. I fired once at a wooden fence near a dumpster, and the sound was so loud that several dogs started to bark, and I quickly ended my practice session. I saw what the many buckshot pellets were capable of doing and was satisfied. I thought about the many holes that had sprayed into the wooden fence and that loud noise as I carried the gun out to the car. Would I be able to do this to a group of people? That thought was pushed away by the image of Rosina and my son being surrounded and intimidated by that band of thugs. My desire for vengeance did not allow my logic to take center stage.

I placed the shotgun in the back seat, still wrapped in the blanket. I soon drove to pick up my wife from her mother's house. We had left our son there with her mom while we drove to find this girl and all her guy friends. We drove up to the house where they were hanging out, but they were gone. A random kid on the street said the group had walked to a fast-food restaurant. We drove there and saw some of them outside as we passed by. We parked about a block away, and I paused for a moment before taking the gun with me. As my hand touched the gun, there was a split second when I hesitated and thought about that fractured wooden fence that had been destroyed by its blast. I considered what that blast would do to a person and the consequences of my walking out of that car with the gun. Then Rosina insisted that I leave the gun in the car. While my fury was no less than it had been immediately after finding out what had happened, I did not want to kill anyone, regardless of what they had done. The other dilemma was that I also didn't want to get jumped, along with Rosina, by this band of teens. Again, my rage suppressed all common sense, and I pushed on without fear of consequence.

We walked over to the restaurant, Rosina just slightly behind me and to my side. The girl was standing outside the restaurant with about five guys of similar age. Her back was turned to me, and the guys spotted me coming before she did.

They seemed to alert the girl to my impending arrival just before we got within steps of her. She was a plump, round-faced teenager. She was wearing a red Fresno State Bulldogs sweater with a red bandana tied into her dark, curly hair. All of her minions were dressed in similar gang-affiliated gear, but based on their youth and sheepish behavior, I suspected they were all wannabes.

While I have never hit a woman and never had any intention of doing her any harm, my fury was focused on her because she was the one who assaulted Rosina. I walked through the surrounding guys and started yelling profanities at her, daring any of the guys with her to look at me challengingly. My hope was that one of them would try to do something so I could redirect my anger physically toward them, but none of them did anything besides watch. Quite surprisingly to me, my wife actually gave a piece of her mind to the girl as well. The girl crouched and covered her head to defend herself as though I were about to start punching her. This reaction looked like a well-rehearsed one, as though she were often a victim herself. She then proceeded to tell us that she was pregnant and to leave her alone. My anger deflated with this new information and behavior, and we walked away. We never had any further problems with this group or anyone else in that neighborhood thereafter. I didn't feel any remorse until years later, when I reflected on all the ways this could have gone wrong.

We could have been arrested, jumped, stabbed, or shot that day. Learning how to control my emotions was one of the first major hurdles I had to overcome. Anger is something that can cause a person to feel justified in doing things they otherwise would never do. Such primitive emotions are evident even in toddlers. One child takes another's toy, and the second retaliates by pushing the first to the ground. Some continue to think this type of behavior is normal if they are not taught otherwise. I was taught from an early age by my step-grandfather that "if somebody messes with you, you need to whoop them." He also said, "If the person is bigger or stronger than you, pick up something heavy and use it to whoop them." I found out many years later, after he passed away, that he had assaulted my grandmother on many occasions and molested my aunt throughout her childhood. One of these occasions, after he had assaulted my grandmother, led to my uncle shooting him in the abdomen and almost killing him. Apparently, he never reported who shot him to the police; I suspect this was out of fear that he would face charges for assault and child molestation once the investigation revealed why he'd been shot.

My familiarity with violence without repercussions is no excuse for considering vengeance when I grabbed the shotgun. But I cannot help but think I had an unconscious bias toward revenge because of what I'd seen as normal behavior my entire life. The "normal" reaction should have been to call the police so they could find that girl and arrest her for assault, instead of me putting our lives and freedom at risk. In retrospect, it is very easy to look at events like this as immature and foolish, but at the time, I felt justified in my actions. It would take a couple more close calls until I finally appreciated how my anger could not only jeopardize my life but also the lives of those I love.

A few months later, we moved out of "Sin City" and into a safer apartment complex a few miles away. We were out of the ghetto, but the ghetto mentality was still part of me. I got into an argument with a guy in our complex over a parking spot. He pulled into the slot I had been waiting for with my blinker on. I honked the horn, only to have him get out of the car to stare me down with his arms held out as if to say, "What are you going to do?" I believe that we can be tempted in many ways, and sometimes our reactions to this temptation can lead to devastating outcomes. This guy was bigger than me, and I was not about to fight with him. The more I allowed my hate and anger to come to the surface, the easier it became to let it out. I stared back at the man as he slowly walked away, glancing sideways at me as he entered the complex. I quickly found another parking slot and caught a glimpse of his apartment. I then ran to my apartment and slammed the door as I entered. Rosina was startled and asked, "What's wrong?" I continued walking to the room and grabbed the gun from under the bed. She persisted, "What are you doing?" I started to explain what had happened, and she stood in my path to the door to stop me. My anger dissipated, and I put the gun away.

Rosina had plans to go out with her friends that day and was concerned that I could be tempted to grab my gun again. Knowing she was not going to be around this time to stop me from doing something foolish, she gave my gun to one of her girlfriends to hold onto until she returned home later that day. When the time came for her to get the gun back, her friend revealed that she was too scared to keep the gun in the house, so she decided to let her boyfriend hold it. When her friend tried to contact her boyfriend to get the gun back, she was unsuccessful. They went over to his house, where he lived with his parents. They found him there, but he told them he had given the gun to somebody else and said he would get the gun back later. When Rosina came home without my gun, I was furious and decided to go over to this guy's house myself. Rosina told me that the guy's parents were home, so despite being upset, she insisted that I be respectful in my efforts.

We pulled up to his house and parked across the street. It was a small house with bars on the windows, a well-kept front yard, and a metal fence around it. We knocked on the door, and the guy answered with a cocky look on his face. I remained quiet to avoid conflict while my wife asked him again for the gun. He responded with attitude, saying he had already told her he didn't have it. This set me off. I demanded that he find the friend he gave my gun to and bring it back.

He said that he couldn't do it, and I became further frustrated and angry. I no longer cared that his parents were home, and I started getting extremely loud. I was on the verge of throwing a punch when his parents came out to see what all the arguing was about. At that point, I started to back off but continued to threaten the guy with his parents standing right there. I warned him that if he did not get my gun, I would be back to deal with him.

Rosina was disappointed with my behavior over a weapon that was not worth fighting for. She had already expressed to me on many previous occasions how much she disliked my having a gun and, in many ways, she probably was happy the gun was gone. That night, I dropped Rosina off at our home, and I stayed at my grandmother's house to cool off.

Later that night, I was awakened by the sound of breaking glass. My first reaction was to run to the front door and look out the window to see what was going on. As I sat up on the couch and was about to stand, Mama yelled out, "Don't get up, stay where you are." Multiple gunshots were then fired into our house. One of the bullets went through the front door and ended up in the wall next to the kitchen. The bullet had passed within inches of where I was sitting on the couch and could have easily ended up in my head instead of the wall if I had leaned forward.

The guy I had verbally assaulted and disrespected in front of his parents attempted to retaliate. He not only did a drive-by on my grandmother's house but also damaged my car parked out front. The initial crash of breaking glass I heard was the sound of a baseball bat smashing my front windshield. Their intention was to make noise by damaging my car, leading me to look out the front door window, only to be shot. Thankfully, my grandmother was there to keep me from getting up.

Immediately after the shooting, I called my wife to let her know what happened. I was quite the idiot at that time and was set on retaliation. I then got her friend's phone number and called her to have the guy and his friends meet me at the corner. I have no idea what I would have done if they showed up. I didn't have my gun, I didn't think of calling any friends with guns for backup, and I didn't even bring so much as a kitchen knife for protection. My blind fury raged so much that I could not even appreciate how lucky I was to be alive and that my grandmother hadn't been shot. Fortunately, nobody showed up as I waited out on the corner like some maniac in the middle of the night. After calming down, I came to realize how foolish I was. I never even laid a hand on the guy; it was simply my anger and my big mouth that put me and my family at risk. Many years later, I decided to dig that bullet out of the wall and keep it as a reminder of how words alone could get you killed in the ghetto.

Several years later, after we had moved away from the neighborhood, one of my wife's friends, whom she had lost contact with over the years, started a relationship with a guy who also had anger issues. They had two children together and were driving somewhere with their kids in the back seat when the guy was cut off by some random person, which led to road rage. Despite having his girlfriend and

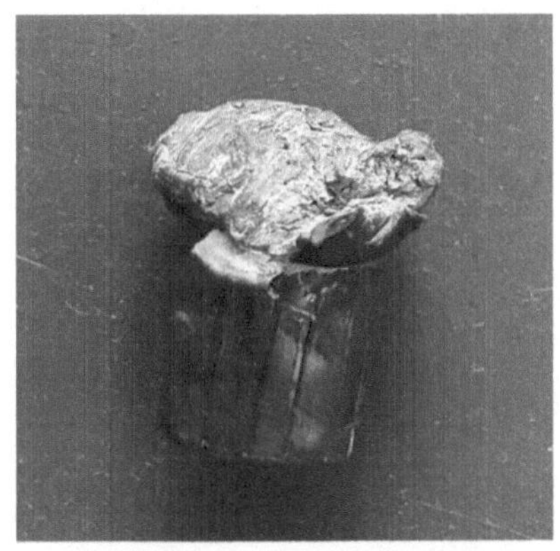

THE ACTUAL BULLET THAT NEARLY HIT MY HEAD WHICH I REMOVED FROM THE WALL IN MAMA'S HOUSE

two kids in the car, he decided to pull in front of the man who initiated the confrontation and slowed to a stop.

The car behind them stopped, too. The guy who was with my wife's friend was carrying a gun. He shot and killed the man in broad daylight, jumped back in the car, and took off. My wife's friend did not report the incident to the police, so when they were caught, he went to prison for life, and she also went to prison as an accessory to murder. Quite a bit is unknown about the situation, but what is certain is that if the guy had not allowed his anger to consume him, he would never have gotten out of the car and killed that man. One bad decision ended one life and destroyed the lives of many others.

Although this was not my story, so many circumstances arose in which I could have easily been in his place and perhaps made the same decision. While I would like to think that I would not have pulled the trigger, I can clearly see the old version of myself behaving in such a reckless manner over being disrespected. Showing anger and responding to evil with evil is allowing others to have power over you. We have control over our emotions, and responding to another's negative actions or behaviors with hostility is not a sign of strength but of weakness.

CHAPTER 9

Lucky

My friend "Lucky" had the kindest soul, and dreamed of a career where he could help others. He was shot and killed on the west side of Fresno, California, while with a group of people outside a nightclub. He was only 19 years old. I was 18, and Rosina was having a baby shower for her pregnancy with our second son, Marcus, that night. For traditional Hispanic baby showers, men typically do not attend, so my wife insisted that I not be present that evening. I picked up my friend George, and we went to a local arcade. We had planned to pick up Lucky that evening, but because he was on the other side of town and I was almost out of gas, I opted not to go get him. Lucky instead went out to a small, crowded nightclub on the west side.

The details concerning the shooter's motive have never been made clear; they often aren't. While at the club that evening, Lucky was shot while standing with a group of people. When the shooter started firing at the crowd, everybody ran. Lucky was hit twice from behind with a shotgun and died instantly. Another man was also shot but sustained non-life-threatening injuries. Lucky was left out on the street for more than 30 minutes before police and paramedics arrived. Quite often on the west side of Fresno, police are much slower to respond to situations like this. Multiple shots being fired are a regular occurrence in the ghetto. Both the police and the people who live in such communities have become used to this. You would think there would already be a ton of police officers not far from this area, given the amount of crime, but for some reason, this is not the case. On the "good" side of Fresno, even a report of shots being fired will result in multiple police units being dispatched to the area. From the perspective of one who has lived in such an area, it can seem like those who are responsible for ensuring the safety of the citizens of Fresno have forgotten about those who live in less affluent areas. Perhaps they feel it is easier to keep the good side good than to improve the "bad" side of town.

Out of all my friends growing up, Lucky was the least likely to have something like this happen to him. He had a really good heart and genuinely wanted to help people by one day becoming a police officer. I often criticized him for this out of my own ignorance, but adding more diversity to neighborhood police forces was probably one of the best ways to improve relationships between the police and the people they are supposed to serve and protect. Lucky was a huge fan of Michael Jordan and the Chicago Bulls and had more basketball skills than most of our friends. Unlike me and some of my other friends, he never looked for trouble and was the least likely in our group to start a fight.

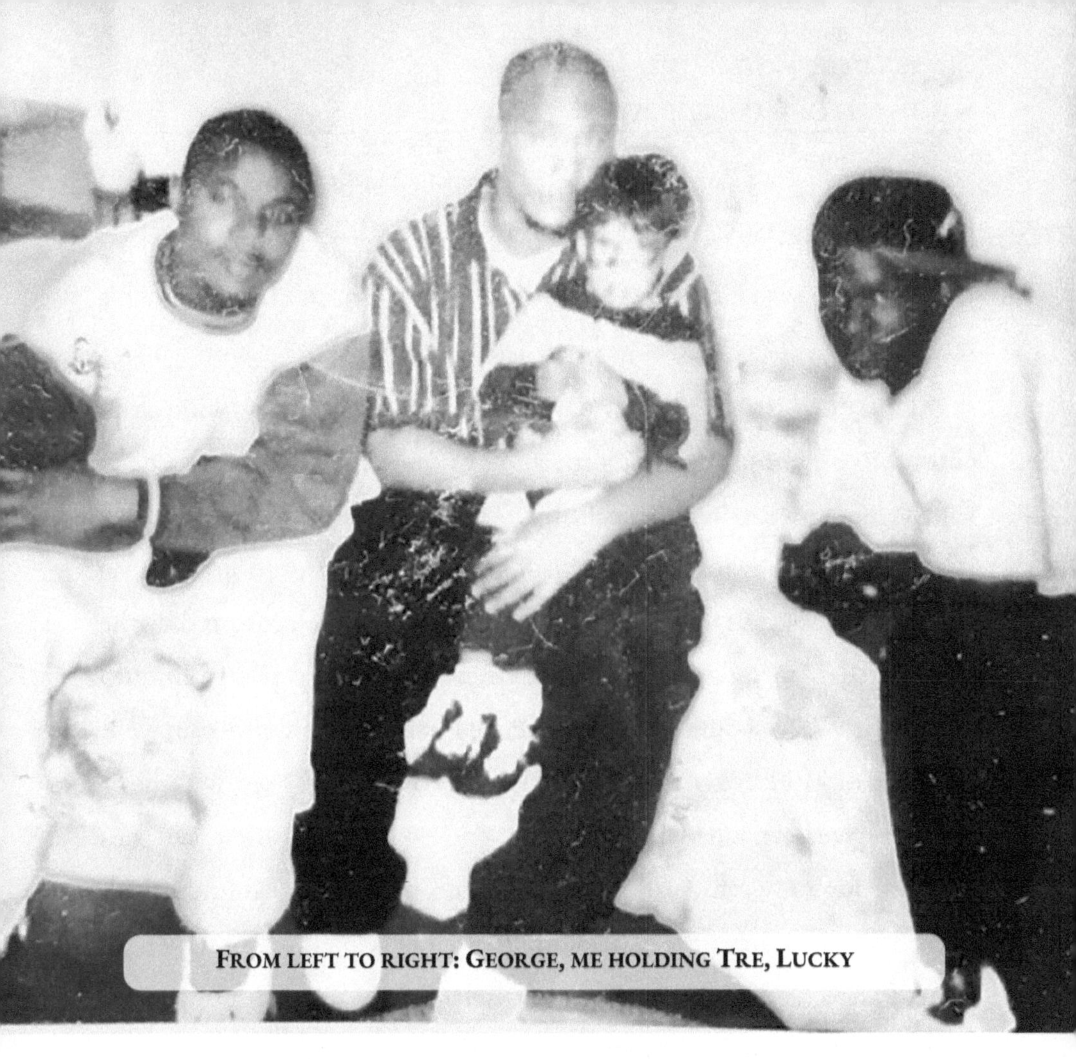

FROM LEFT TO RIGHT: GEORGE, ME HOLDING TRE, LUCKY

I find it hard to understand how those of us who were constantly getting into trouble managed to escape the fate that Lucky met. My faith and spirit were troubled by this. How could this happen to him when there are others like me who had been in so many worse situations and harmed so many others? It would not be until years later that I would begin to understand some of God's truths, which today bring me comfort. For us to truly love God and to love others, we must have free will. Without free will, we are only robots following a script. Free will means that we have the freedom to choose between good and evil. As a consequence, anyone can fall victim to the evil acts of others. This world is not Heaven—far from it. This world is temporary, and I believe that Lucky is now with God. This brings me comfort because I know that his family and all of his friends will one day be reunited.

I attended the wake a few days after his death. I was working as an automotive technician at the time and got off work early to see Lucky for the last time at the funeral home. The family chose a funeral home not very far from where he was killed. I drove past the location where he was shot and tried to imagine how it all went down. I felt tortured by the thought that Lucky would still have been alive if I had picked him up that night. What would I have done if I had been there when it all went down? Could I have prevented Lucky's death if I had been with him? Could I have been killed if I had been there? So many different scenarios went through my mind as I drove, and like a time warp, I found myself parked out in front of the funeral home with little memory of how I got there. I arrived a bit early and was somewhat afraid to get out of the car. It was my first time experiencing the death of someone close to me, and I was anxious about going into the funeral home alone. After ten minutes of waiting to see if anybody I knew would show up, I finally decided to go in by myself.

The funeral home was a single-story building with a concrete path leading straight from the sidewalk to a set of large wooden double doors. I entered the lobby, where there were signs posted for other viewings. I became anxious when I didn't immediately see my friend's name, but one of the greeters approached me and asked, "Which family are you here for?" *"What an interesting way to address* visitors," I thought. "The loved one who has passed is who you are there to see, but I suspect in this business, asking the visitor to say the name of the departed may be enough to start the flood of emotions far too early. Saying you are there for the family is, in part, true, but more so, you are there to see a loved one for the last time." Lucky was in one of the rooms toward the back of the building. I was shown the way and felt as though my stomach dropped and my legs grew heavy as I slowly walked to his room.

A sign outside his room had his last name on it. The open casket was straight ahead, at the back of the room, with basic white chairs lined in rows on each side of a center aisle. My eyes immediately moved across the room to see that there were no other family members or friends there. I could see from the door that the casket was open, but I did not allow my gaze to look directly at him until I had first looked around the room. After being certain there was no one else there yet, I slowly walked in.

Lucky was one of my best friends, but I was afraid of what his family would think. Did the family know I wasn't with him the night he died? Did they know that we talked about picking him up to go with us to the arcade, but we decided to go without him? Would they know that if I had picked him up that night, he might never have gone to the club with another group of friends where he was killed?

I slowly walked down the center aisle toward my friend and felt uneasy, as though I was doing something wrong. I looked behind me to see if I was still alone. I was. I placed my hand on Lucky's chest and was shocked when there was significant give. It was too soft, and it felt padded. He was shot in the back of the head and torso, so I imagined that part of his chest was missing. I moved my hand back to the side of the casket. Unlike on television, where deceased people often look as they did when they were alive, Lucky did not look like himself. His face was swollen around the mouth, and his skin looked as though it had been painted in places, the contours of his forehead and cheek slightly off. I touched his hands, which were crossed over one another, and they were incredibly cold and hard. I whispered to Lucky that I was sorry for not picking him up that night. Tears began to well up as I thought about how things might have been different if I had made the trip. All of his dreams were taken from him by some idiot with a gun. Family and other friends started to arrive, and the small ceremony began, with music playing and words shared about the good times. Many tears were shed.

His mother, who was utterly devastated by the loss of her son, sat in the front with the look of a person who had a part of her soul ripped away. She stared forward, slightly slumped in the chair with a handful of balled-up tissues. She appeared numb from the shock of it all. She had given up wiping tracks of tears on her face. A parent should never have to bury their own child. No parent ever thinks they will be in such a position, and when it happens, there can be no good way to prepare for it.

Joseph Stalin, the former leader of the communist Soviet Union, once said, "A single death is a tragedy; a million deaths, a statistic." People like Stalin and Hitler took advantage of this unfortunate truth. It is difficult to comprehend something as horrible as the death of a million people, or even a hundred. Some can easily turn a blind eye to tragedies because they often hear nothing more than statistics being reported in the media. Here in America, in some of our very own neighborhoods, people are being killed every day, often over something as trivial as the color of clothes or for standing in the wrong place. You hear about this on the news somewhere between the discussion of the weather forecast and the critics' choice for best movie. Murders are no longer major news unless they involve a mass shooting, but even then, they often become politicized for a few days before fading away.

For the family and friends of the victims, their lives are forever changed, but for most others, there is very little impact. Most people have never lost a family member or a friend to violence, so the emotional tie to such tragic events is often lacking. Even those who live in communities regularly affected by such tragedies have become desensitized to the violence. For many, there is probably a stronger emotional reaction to those depressing commercials about abandoned dogs or cats at risk of euthanasia. Quite often, people are more mortified by a story discussing the death of "man's best friend" than man himself. While I, too, may no longer be surprised when frequent murders in the poorest neighborhoods are briefly mentioned in the news, these stories do make me reflect on the loss I felt when Lucky was murdered. Life without my friend went on, but I was forever changed by his loss. I had started my own family and had placed myself in far more dangerous situations than Lucky had ever been in. It didn't seem fair that I was the one still alive. Survivor's guilt is a very real phenomenon that causes some to fall into a rut. I had an obligation to my family to make something of the life I had. A person can only have so many close calls. It was time for me to learn from my mistakes and move forward. My opportunity to go to college would be wasted if I continued to put myself in dangerous situations. This turning point in my life was when I finally walked away from the lifestyle that would have eventually ruined me.

CHAPTER 10

A Way Out

It was unconventional and spontaneous, the way it happened. We were both sitting on the couch watching television, and the thought just crossed my mind: *Should we get married?* We already had two kids, and we obviously loved each other. I looked at her and said, "Why aren't we married?" Rosina had a somewhat surprised look on her face and shrugged her shoulders. Her facial expression changed slightly, implying she was thinking, *My point exactly.* We contemplated taking the leap right then, but got married in her brother's backyard the next day. It was all short notice, though we had even contemplated getting married the same day. Ultimately, we thought it would be appropriate to give our families some notice. It was a small ceremony that cost no more than $500, which was partially contributed by Rosina's siblings. We had very few material possessions, but our love made up for this in abundance. We both wanted to provide a better future for our children than our own. This was our chance to find a way out of the life expected of teenage parents.

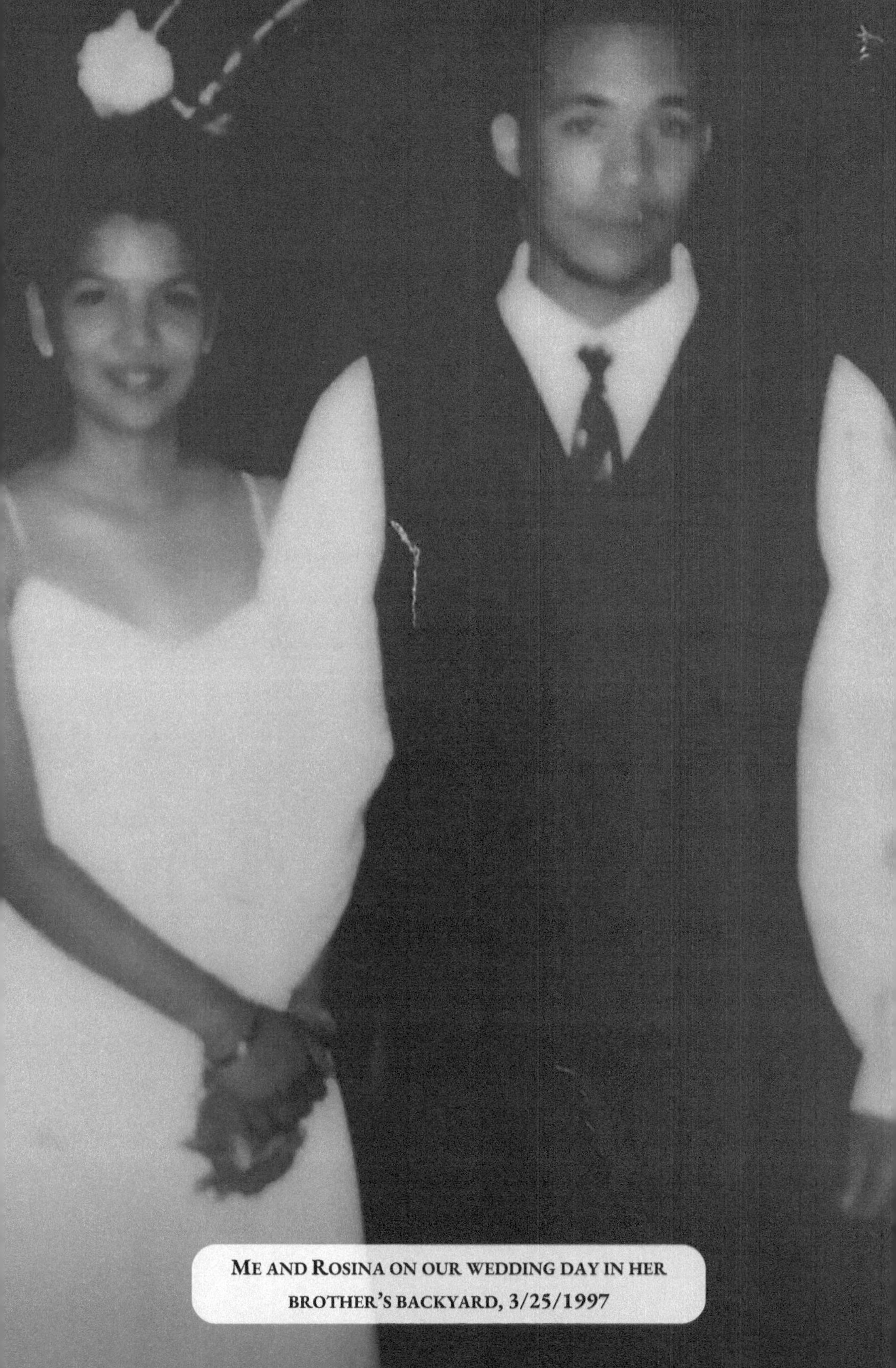

Me and Rosina on our wedding day in her brother's backyard, 3/25/1997

Rosina graduated from high school a year before me and worked in various factories and department stores for a little over a year before deciding to attend a junior college for an associate's degree in medical assisting. It was a fast way to make more money for our family. She continued to work while attending night school. I also worked at various jobs while still attending Ted C. Wills Restart High School. One day, while dropping off my home studies assignment with my teacher, Mr. Pitt, I was approached by one of the school counselors, Mr. Henry Ray. Mr. Ray asked me to sit down with him at his desk to "discuss some things." I had been cheating in my home studies class by copying answers out of the book, so my first thought was that I had somehow been caught. Having been interviewed on a few occasions in the past by security guards and police regarding acts for which I had been completely guilty, I learned to keep my mouth shut until asked a question and then calmly lie and deny any wrongdoing. My previous experience with counselors at my other high school always seemed to focus on all the problems in my life; these meetings were never pleasant, and I expected this one to be more of the same.

Mr. Ray was middle-aged at the time, and I thought he resembled Malcolm X. He had a very calm demeanor, with a short afro and a sport coat. After I sat down, preparing to be lectured about how I had screwed up, he said in his very characteristic and moderately shrill voice, "James, what the heck is your problem?" *Oh boy,* I thought, *here we go.* Apparently, he had wanted to speak with me for some time, and I had avoided him for long enough. "I hear you just had a child, and you're spending so much time working that you're barely going to graduate on time. Is that all you want to do with your life?" Although he came across a little rough and frustrated, throughout high school, no counselor or teacher had ever seemed to care about my future plans. That being said, I was ditching most of the time and didn't show the slightest bit of interest in the future to anybody. Despite my negative attitude, Mr. Ray was determined to get me talking.

I defiantly responded to Mr. Ray. "What do you expect me to do? My grandma lives off her disability check, and she still receives welfare and food stamps for me. We don't have money for college applications, let alone college." Mr. Ray quickly stopped me before I had a chance to say another word. "Whoa, whoa, whoa, what makes you think you need to have money to go to college? For kids like you who don't have money for college, financial aid, scholarships, and even loans exist to help you get your education and become whatever it is you want to be."

I was immediately humbled and completely subdued by what he told me. I had no idea students, like myself, who were not only financially disadvantaged but also average at best academically could ever go to college. Mr. Ray then asked me, "Do you have any idea what you want to do?"

It had probably been since early middle school that I had last spoken to anyone about my dream of becoming a doctor. I shared this with him, and he said, "Here's what you're going to do: fill out this paperwork with your grandma's financial information, and go to Fresno State University's Equal Opportunity Program office and ask for Wayne Byrd. Your grades are not good enough to go straight to Fresno State on your own, but this person can look beyond your grades and give you a chance. You are going to go to Fresno State and become whatever it is you want to be."

I did indeed meet with Wayne Byrd, who looked over my application and spoke with me for some time. He came across as genuinely interested in who I was and what my goals were. The fact that I was working full-time while in high school and had a young child to support did not discourage him from giving me a chance to attend Fresno State. At the time, I knew this was something significant, but it wasn't until six years later, as I approached graduation from Fresno State (yes, working full-time while in school did extend how long it took to graduate from college) and had been accepted to medical school at the University of California, Los Angeles (UCLA), that I truly appreciated how critical a role both Mr. Ray and Mr. Byrd had in my life. They both looked beyond my obvious disadvantages and somehow recognized my potential. I later returned to their offices with a package for each of them that contained thank-you cards and a copy of my acceptance letter to UCLA's medical school. I was the first student to graduate from that high school to go on to medical school, so Mr. Ray was very excited to hear the news.

I often think back to where I was when Mr. Ray pulled me aside and decided to invest his time in me. I looked like a thug, was a horrible student, and showed very little interest in academics. What magical gift does one possess to see the potential of another person who can't even see his or her own potential? I never asked why he chose to help me, but I suspect the most likely answer is that there was nothing particularly special about me. Mr. Ray helped every student with whom he sat down, and if you roll the dice long enough, eventually you are going to win a few times. It sounds much better to speculate that I was chosen for some reason, but the reality is that there are so many kids out there who can become the next doctor, lawyer, or politician; all they need is an opportunity. Most are never offered that opportunity because they are judged based on what others think of them. If more counselors and teachers were like Mr. Ray, many more students from underserved areas could have stories very similar to mine. My successes all started with a small nudge in the right direction from someone who believed in me. The world can use more Mr. Rays in it. I lost track of him over the years after my old high school closed and have been unable to find him. Mr. Ray lived a life inspiring others to be the best they could be, but he did not leave a large footprint on the internet. I pray that he knew how much his selfless work changed my life.

Getting me into college was a huge accomplishment on its own, but getting me to succeed presented a whole different set of challenges. The financial challenge was always the priority because of my obligation to my family. When I started going to Fresno State, my wife and I were both working full-time. I worked full-time as an auto technician and part-time at a toy store. I usually tried to arrange my school schedule so that all classes fell on Tuesdays and Thursdays. These were my two days off from work.

My wife is an amazing woman who has been incredibly supportive. Over the years, she managed to work full-time while taking care of the house, the kids, and me. Even though I have always done everything I could for the good of our family, she has truly been the foundation that has kept our family strong. When the kids needed something for school or had to go to the doctor, she was always there. Without her, I could have never worked and attended school full-time.

Given that I spent most of my first two years of high school ditching and the last two years playing catch-up, I wasn't completely prepared for higher education. While I was thankful for the opportunity to go straight to college from high school, I was clearly not ready. Math and English were by far my two most neglected subjects in high school, so when I got to Fresno State, I purposely avoided those classes for my first semester. I did fairly well that semester, obtaining a 3.4 GPA, but I knew that I would soon have to struggle through math and English the following semester. Math, in particular, had been neglected for so long that I didn't even remember how to add fractions when I got to college. I had to take a screening math and English placement test, and I failed both of them horribly. My poor performance meant I had to take a year of prerequisite math and a semester of prerequisite English before being allowed to move on to the standard college-level math and English required for graduation. In addition to my academic challenges as a full-time student, I was still working full-time, and Rosina was pregnant with our second child, Marcus.

It didn't take long for me to realize that if I was going to make it through college, I would need help. A free tutoring center at Fresno State gave me the opportunity to catch up, but asking for help and being so far behind was embarrassing. Most fourth graders were more advanced in their math skills than I was, and being a pre-med college student with this level of deficiency was unheard of. My first visit to the tutoring center was quite intimidating. The Education Building was located in the back of the university's property, away from all the science buildings; this was a good thing because I was terrified I would run into another pre-med student who would find out my secret.

I was raised being told how smart I was by my grandmother, so I did have a strong sense of confidence and pride. I was quite bright growing up, but no matter how smart I thought I was, once I got behind in math, it felt impossible to catch up. The system in America often passes students along regardless of how far behind they are. I made it through the system but then had to swallow my pride, humble myself, and reveal to another person that I was performing at the math level of a second grader. I walked into the tutoring center just after lunch and met with one of the math tutors. Also a student, he was a math major who was quite bright but not very patient. He looked at me as though I were playing a practical joke when I shared that I was taking physics but did not remember how to add fractions. My first day sitting in trigonometry-based physics included a rapid-fire review of "simple trigonometry," in which the young professor with horn-rimmed glasses stated, "We won't waste too much of your time going over this." My tutor looked me up and down with disbelief and asked if I truly didn't know, as though he needed confirmation that I wasn't joking before proceeding to teach simple math. Although we had a painful start, I was a fast learner, and since I had known much of this material at one point, I quickly picked it up again. This allowed us to move forward and build upon these basic math skills and then begin learning algebra and trigonometry. Not having mastered this material before taking physics did put me at a disadvantage, but I was able to catch up through countless hours of late-night studying. I often took my books to work so that I could study during my lunch breaks. With all the tutoring and studying, I was able to finish both semesters of physics with a "B." Although I had set goals of acing all of my pre-med requirements, I didn't beat myself up over it.

For many, college is an exhilarating experience filled with new adventures. It's often their first time being independent. For me, that independence began when I was 15, after finding out I was going to be a father. Undergraduate life can be enjoyable when there's time to balance academic and extracurricular activities, but for me, undergrad was hell. To pay the bills, I worked up to three jobs while attending Fresno State, making my time there far from enjoyable. During my second semester, I worked my two jobs and added a part-time position at a hatchery. That semester was challenging not only because of the heavy workload from these jobs but also because it was my first time taking math and English at the college level. I took only three classes that semester, scheduling them in the evening to keep my work schedule open for forty hours a week at the auto shop. I worked weekends at the toy store during the day and usually squeezed in a few graveyard shifts at the hatchery to make extra money to cover the new expenses from the birth of our middle son, Marcus. My wife worked full-time until the day she went into labor and took only a few weeks off after his birth. Still, living paycheck to paycheck, this loss of income made it challenging to keep our heads above water.

The stress of working three jobs, caring for a newborn, and attending college became too much for me to handle. Of all the stressors at the time, the hatchery job became my breaking point. The hatchery was a large industrial facility where chicks were hatched, sorted, and then sent to other areas of the facility to be fed and allowed to mature before being used for food. My simple job duties there involved working the graveyard shift, putting on coveralls, and standing at an assembly line where I spent the entire night dumping trays full of freshly hatched chicks onto a conveyor belt. The chicks were then evaluated as they rolled up the conveyor belt to be sorted. Those that were dead or did not appear healthy enough to survive were thrown on the floor and disposed of at the end of the shift. The entire process felt like a nightmare; my body ached from the repetitive motion of grabbing and repeatedly dumping the heavy trays. I was covered in a yellow dust from the freshly hatched eggs, which worked its way into every exposed part of my body and even into my lungs. Dead and barely alive chicks littered the ground, and the entire time, their cries of "cheep, cheep, cheep" overwhelmed my ears.

While on the line, I was afraid of stepping on the chicks that had been thrown on the ground, so I tried to avoid taking large steps by shuffling my feet as I moved. A few times I accidentally stepped on some of the chicks, some of which were still alive. To this day, I can still feel and hear the bones cracking, sending chills up my spine. During my lunch break, I was too disgusted to eat. The dust particles left a foul taste in my mouth, and the constant cheeping could be heard from the break room, so it was too distracting to study on my breaks as I did at my other jobs. At the end of the shift, I had to sweep up all of the chicks from the floor and then put them into a large dumpster. Some of the chicks, deformed from congenital abnormalities, were still clinging to life. The image of these dead and barely alive chicks still haunts me; I lasted at this job for just over two weeks before quitting.

That semester in college, while working at the hatchery, I also walked away from the university. I did not withdraw or request to have an incomplete; I simply stopped attending and received an entire semester of Fs. Time to study was non-existent. I slept between jobs and during lunch breaks, and I was spending very little time at home with my family. My life had become a blur, with no time to focus or excel at anything. My priority was to support my family, but by being stretched so thin, I was jeopardizing my health, job performance, academic drive, and my ability to be a husband and father. By letting go of my school responsibilities, I was able to regain control of one of the most under-appreciated assets I possessed: my time. Although my education was important to me, at the time we needed financial security to survive, so I had to put this aspect of my life on hold. I spent more time with my family and improved my focus and dedication to work. My work performance was recognized by my manager at the auto shop, and I was promoted to service manager. I was nineteen years old and the youngest service manager they had ever had at that shop—or in the entire region.

Possessing the drive to succeed does help in creating opportunities, but I feel that these opportunities could have been lost if I had allowed my failures to become my focus. Dropping out of college was a huge hit to my ego, and I felt like a failure. I was embarrassed and didn't share my feelings with anyone. Instead of allowing my failure to become the focus of my life, I decided to concentrate on excelling in other areas where I had control. I did not abandon my hopes and dreams of becoming a physician, but I realized that if I could regain more time to focus, I could try again when conditions were more favorable. I quit early in the semester, shortly after leaving the horrible job at the hatchery. I started making more money as a service manager and also arranged my work schedule so I could control my working hours. I worked weekends only at the toy store and planned to quit that job and return to school the following semester, once my wife completed her maternity leave and returned to work.

After Rosina started working again, I quit my weekend job and returned to school. Rosina also decided to go back to school, but she wanted to minimize the long-term struggle by attending a trade school for medical assisting. With control of my schedule, I was able to dedicate time to studying, and my grades began to improve. I sought help from tutors and classmates whenever the material was challenging. I was still behind in math and English, but after completing remedial classes and putting in extra time relearning the basics with tutors, I was able to excel in all areas. Learning how to study efficiently was important for me because of the limited time I had compared to other students. Working full-time was my substitute for extracurricular activities.

Once my grades and confidence improved, I sought the advice of a pre-med advisor. I scheduled an appointment to discuss the direction I should take with my classes, when to take the Medical College Admission Test (MCAT), and when to apply to medical school. I went into the meeting excited about the future, but left feeling deflated and uncertain about the possibility of being accepted into medical school. The advisor told me that if I were going to get into medical school, I would need to cut back on work hours in order to focus fully on school. She believed that working full-time would make it extremely difficult to excel academically. My wife and I were both working full-time to support our family, but we were barely keeping our heads above water. We lived paycheck to paycheck without a safety net. The advisor suggested that I consider an alternative career path instead of medical school. "Why don't you consider teaching instead?" I left that session uncertain and frustrated. Even though there was some truth in the advice, what is true for most does not have to be true for all. One of the biggest problems that tarnished my application was the full semester of Fs from when I temporarily left school. She had never seen a student with that many Fs be accepted into medical school, even if it was only one semester. Some universities allowed grade replacement if a failed class was repeated, but Fresno State did not. My academic record was forever tarnished.

While my path was unusual and difficult, it was not impossible. I did consider other alternatives for a short period of time, but I couldn't let go of my dream. Fear of failure stops many people from even trying to accomplish something that may seem too challenging. What I knew for certain was that if I did not try, my chance for success would be zero. I worked hard and learned the material for all of my classes by studying late at night while my family slept. I improved my GPA by earning A's in most of my classes, making that horrible semester of F's look less representative of who I was. I was determined not to let my history define who I would become. I learned from my failures and worked hard to build a better future for my family. While I remained focused on my goals, my accomplishments motivated me, but they were not enough to sustain me. A spiritual heaviness was present as I pressed on with my microsuccesses. I had stopped praying for years because I prioritized everything else over God. I had been pulled from the darkness by His hand but then continued to believe that my success came from my efforts alone. I had been blessed with a wife, children, and opportunities that I felt were undeserved, yet none of these things felt sufficient. It was God's grace that brought me out of the darkness. My spiritual journey would not be fully recognized until years later, but even though I did not acknowledge God's help during this period of my life, like any good parent, He was still there with me.

CHAPTER 11

Desperation for God

A deep fear and the feeling that my heart had dropped into my stomach, gripped me in a split second as I braked quickly at the light on my way to Fresno State for one of my afternoon classes. I immediately looked in the rearview mirror after stopping suddenly to avoid hitting the car in front of me, only to see the pickup truck rapidly approaching from behind. I did not have time to react, and the reality that death might have come for me at that very moment terrified me. This fear forced me to think about what would happen to me when my time came to draw my last breath. I had no serious injuries besides some neck and back pain, but my car was totaled. The driver had insurance, and life went on. Cars come and go, but I suspect it was this experience that served as a wake-up call, opening my eyes to look for what was missing in my life.

Several days later, during finals week, I really found God. I had shaken off the nerves from the accident and felt pretty confident that I was ready to handle all my finals. Life was busy with full-time work and school while being a husband and a father. I had figured out a system to use my time efficiently for studying and was on a path to get a 4.0 that semester. Despite all the positive things in my life, there was a darkness that followed me. Even when everything seemed to be going well (minus the near-death experience), an emptiness I could not shake persisted. I could not shed the guilt that I carried from the wrongs in my past, and I spent every day in fear that these sins would be repaid to me without warning. If I had died the day of the crash, what would have happened to me? I was desperately seeking freedom from this fear, wondering when the day of reckoning would come. I had a debt that was quite large and had no idea how to repay it.

One day, I was in one of the common areas of the university where many students found comfortable places to cram in last-minute study sessions. I was on a break and decided to relax and look around the room. Many students worked in isolation with their heads buried in books. A few were taking breaks like I was, and one group of students was sitting in a small circle with what looked like Bibles. I was a bit too far away to hear what they were saying, but I was intrigued. I casually collected my things, packed my backpack, and walked toward the exit door in the group's direction. As I passed, one of the students made eye contact with me and smiled. He waved and got up to say hello. His name was Tyrone, and he invited me to join their Bible study. I had not thought much about God for some time, and being a biology major and pre-med student, part of me felt that any person of faith would not want anything to do with me. Despite this, I sat down, introduced myself to the group, and listened.

The group was diverse, well-spoken, kind, and well-versed in the Bible. They also appeared to be students from various majors and, like me, were on top of their studies and still made time for a Bible study. I was invited to participate in future Bible studies, and unlike offers from other friends to go to the bar or out to eat (which I usually declined), I felt a tug in my heart to accept this one. I was still working full-time and taking a full semester of classes, so outside of my obligations, all other time was spent at home with my family. I bought my first Bible before starting the next Bible study and began studying the Gospels in my free time. I felt as though this studying was very different from the studying for my pre-med classes. I felt like the Word of God was changing my heart and causing me to worry about my salvation. I had a dark history, and for many years, I thought of myself as a bad person. I was trying to be a good person for my family, but not even my family was enough to cause real change from within. When I read about repentance, I took this very seriously and had already turned away from my old ways, but the part about baptism and forgiveness of sins was what really got my attention. I had a loose understanding of God's ways before I started reading the Bible, but I was scared that someday all of my sins would come back to haunt me. When I found out that baptism with repentance could give me a clean slate, I became desperate for this solution.

A story in the Bible is told in three separate books: Matthew 9:20–22, Mark 5:27–34, and Luke 8:43–48. In it, a woman was desperate for help because she had been bleeding for twelve years. She had seen many doctors, and none were able to cure her. At that time, Jesus had already gained a reputation for performing miracles, so whenever He was seen, large crowds would gather. When this woman heard that Jesus was in town, she had to make her way to Him. She had such strong faith that if she could only touch His clothing, she believed she would be healed. The problem was that at that time, women were considered unclean when they were bleeding, and they were not allowed to come in contact with others during menstruation. She was living as an outcast, as were those who had leprosy. For her to risk going out into a crowd, pushing through others, and then touching Jesus was a huge risk, but she was so desperate to be saved that her faith drove her to find Him. This woman pushed through the crowd to make her way to Jesus, where she was able to reach out and touch part of His clothing and was immediately healed. I think of this story when I consider the desperation I felt when I was constantly worried about my life and my future, despite making positive progress in work and school. I was spiritually bleeding for years, and I was afraid that my past was going to come back to punish me for the wrongs I had done to others in my youth. For many years, I carried a burden of guilt and shame that kept me spiritually isolated. Once I discovered that the cure was to turn away from my old ways and to wash away all the wrongs of my past with baptism, I was laser-focused on making this happen.

At the next Bible study, I met the church's pastor, Dan. Within a few minutes of starting the Bible study, I cut to the chase and shared with the group that I needed to be baptized. The group was happy to hear this, but they wanted to go over some parts of the Bible with me in detail to make sure I was ready for this commitment. I had already read these chapters and didn't need any further explanation; my fear and desperation for forgiveness of my sins and God's salvation were what drove me. My worries about karma coming back to hurt me were not taught in the Bible; rather, there is an emphasis on repentance and forgiveness. I insisted that I be baptized immediately. Further attempts were made to get me to slow my roll, but I threatened to find another group or a local church to do the deed for me. I had attended only a few church services before becoming completely committed to this as my path to washing away the sins of my past. These sins haunted me, and I felt it was my only means of escape.

Although I was ready to venture out on my own to be baptized, I listened to their advice and went over a few more lessons in the Bible. I ran at such high speed in desperation to be saved that my wife was left behind. I let her know what I was doing, but she did not feel that same desire to proceed as quickly as I did. Rosina was raised in the Catholic Church, and although Catholics believe in baptism, their tradition tends to offer baptism to infants. Rosina had been baptized as an infant, and she did not have any desire to relive the experience. She had not attended the Bible studies that I had participated in, so she also felt a bit left out. She also did not have the kind of past wrongdoing hanging over her head as I did. I became extremely zealous about what the Bible said and started pointing out areas I felt she should consider regarding the way we worship and serve God. This did not go over well.

Religion started to become a topic that led to arguments, and I became disheartened because I thought I was doing the right thing, but the most important part of my life, outside of God, was now being compromised. This animosity was pushing us apart, so I kept my feelings about Jesus and the Bible to myself, feeling like a bad father and husband for not being able to share this part of my life with my family. Despite my passion for God, I was under the greatest spiritual attack and was losing the battle. Fear of losing my family eventually silenced me on religion. While I maintained my faith internally, my isolation from church and from sharing this aspect of my life regularly with others led to spiritual weakness. I stopped going to church and tried to maintain a loose connection with God through prayer and reading the Bible when I had the chance. In Luke 8:10–15, Jesus tells the parable of the seeds scattered in different areas and what happens to the seed depending on where it falls. The seed represents the Word of God, and the various locations where the seed falls represent the people who hear the word. I was like the seed that fell on rocky ground: quickly accepted but without deep roots. In a time of testing, there was no strong foundation, so I fell away.

As college and work became more time-consuming, my spiritual growth was stagnant. I was too early in my faith and could not see that it was not about religion but about the unconditional love of Jesus for all people that conquers all negativity. I became so fixated on the details of religion and the practices of others that I lost sight of what was in my own heart. Jesus said that the greatest commandment is to love God with all your heart, soul, and mind, but equally important is to love your neighbor as yourself. The Gospels of Matthew, Mark, and Luke all emphasize this important lesson from Jesus, but I did not listen. By making overzealous attempts to correct the differences in others, I ignored what Jesus taught and, like a greedy miser, kept the treasure of God's love all to myself for many years. It was not until more than twenty-five years later, when I had a spiritual awakening after my wife started studying the Bible with some of her friends, that we were able to come together on common ground about Jesus and the teachings of the Bible.

I still had God's Word in my heart, but I shifted my time away from church activities and became locked in on my goal of becoming a physician. Focused on academics and the next big step of getting into medical school, I started preparing for the dreaded MCAT. My downfall was that I focused on performing well in each college class, but as soon as that class was completed, I moved on to the next without attempting to retain the information for the long term. I did hold on to some critical aspects and general principles, but what I failed to prepare for was the huge comprehensive test that would bring back all the material I thought I would never need to recall again. The MCAT is a combination of biology, general chemistry, organic chemistry, biochemistry, physics, and English, all in one session. Not only did I need to relearn all the material I dumped from my brain to make space for the next semester's classes, but I was also not strong at taking standardized tests. Somehow, I managed to get accepted to Fresno State through the EOP without having to take the Scholastic Aptitude Test (SAT) or American College Test (ACT). While this opportunity was appreciated, I was unprepared when the time came for my first real standardized test.

My first attempt at the MCAT was a failure. I was working full-time and taking a full semester of classes while studying for the MCAT, and I ended up performing below average in every category. I had plans to apply to medical school the following year, so I had another opportunity to take the MCAT again, but the next time, I was prepared to attack with a different strategy: I took a lighter load of classes that semester, saved all my vacation time from work for MCAT preparation, and obtained a scholarship for an MCAT preparation course. I followed an intense schedule of studying six days a week for eight hours a day and took all of the available practice tests. When the time came for the real test, I was much more prepared. Despite all the hard work, I still struggled with test anxiety and my lack of experience taking standardized tests over the previous years. I did improve my scores, but only marginally. I had to accept my below-average performance and move on with the application process for medical school.

I was terrified that I would apply to medical school, like many of my other pre-med friends over the years, and not get accepted. I decided to apply to as many medical schools as I could. I also acquired applications for medical schools with a high acceptance rate outside of the United States as a backup plan. I even spoke with a recruiter from a medical school in the Caribbean who made the idea of medical school overseas sound quite appealing; he bragged that students spent days studying on the beach. Many brilliant and well-trained physicians left the United States for various reasons to complete their medical school training abroad, but this strategy does put them at a disadvantage because they compete with those who have trained in the United States when applying for residency. Although I knew I could be at a disadvantage later in the process, I was willing to utilize any path necessary to achieve my goal of becoming a physician. I even considered schools in Mexico, even though I did not speak Spanish. In the end, I feel my attitude and tenacity opened many doors for me. I would have happily accepted any opportunity to achieve my goal of becoming a physician; this lack of reservation and appreciation for any program that gave me a chance had a positive impact on the way I was perceived by those who interviewed me.

Despite having only mediocre MCAT scores and a failed second semester in college, I was able to get into medical school. My overall GPA with a positive trend, a unique personal statement, and life experiences helped me overcome my areas of weakness. I received interviews from many of the medical schools I applied to and had multiple acceptances. My dream program was UCLA, and it was my final interview for the year. My most memorable interviewer was Dr. Isabel-Jones, a prominent pediatric cardiologist who was the first African-American woman to join this specialty in the United States. She really took time to get to know me and was able to look beyond some of the areas of weakness in my application that I am certain raised eyebrows among the other faculty on the admissions committee. Many years later, I was told by a member of the committee who was present when Dr. Isabel-Jones discussed my application that she stood her ground and fought for me to be given a chance. Despite my low MCAT scores, likely the lowest scores in my class, and a semester of Fs, I was given the opportunity to pursue my dream of becoming a physician at UCLA.

Before I was officially told that I had been awarded a spot, Dr. Isabel-Jones invited me to a dinner that was to occur that evening after my interview for the students who had been accepted to the program. I had just interviewed that day and felt great about how everything went but had no official confirmation that I was accepted. At the dinner, I brought my wife, and we met many of the other students and faculty, who were a bit surprised that I was invited to this event. A few said, "If you are here, you definitely have a spot." Dr. Isabel-Jones had only met me that day, and I will be forever grateful that she took a chance and advocated for me. If there was one moment in my life when I felt like an imposter, it was then.

Besides its fantastic reputation, UCLA was close to home and had a great network of resources for students with families. The cost of living in Los Angeles is quite high, but the university offered married student housing, which was subsidized, with spacious three-bedroom apartments only fifteen minutes away from the medical school. My kids were able to attend great public schools that were a short walk from our apartment, and there was a great network of like-minded, goal-oriented families who were our neighbors and friends.

One of the nice things about going to medical school that made it feel a bit less intimidating was that everyone started on a level playing field. No one had been through the medical school curriculum, so despite their intimidating Ivy League backgrounds, we were all navigating uncharted territory. Unlike my rough start in undergrad, medical school was a great experience. For the first time, I no longer had to work full-time while in school. I was able to take out loans to cover my expenses and just focus on school. The material could be challenging at times, but it was enjoyable. Some describe the volume of material one has to learn in medical school as taking a drink of water from a fire hydrant, but I disagree. If you put in the time to spread out a large volume of material over the semester, rather than try to cram it all in during the last week before the test, it becomes not just tolerable but, dare I say, fun. I enjoyed being a student again. All of my effort was now on getting the most out of medical school so that I could become the best doctor I could be. This journey strengthened my work ethic and my commitment to my career, but my heart became hardened to God's presence as I increasingly believed that it was through my works alone that my goals were coming to fruition. Sometimes our success in worldly accomplishments can push us away from God, and if and when it all comes crashing down, the loss of status or possessions may lead to drastic actions such as substance abuse or even suicide. It is best to be humble and be grateful for what we have, but always stay focused on what is most important: our relationship with God and serving Him first.

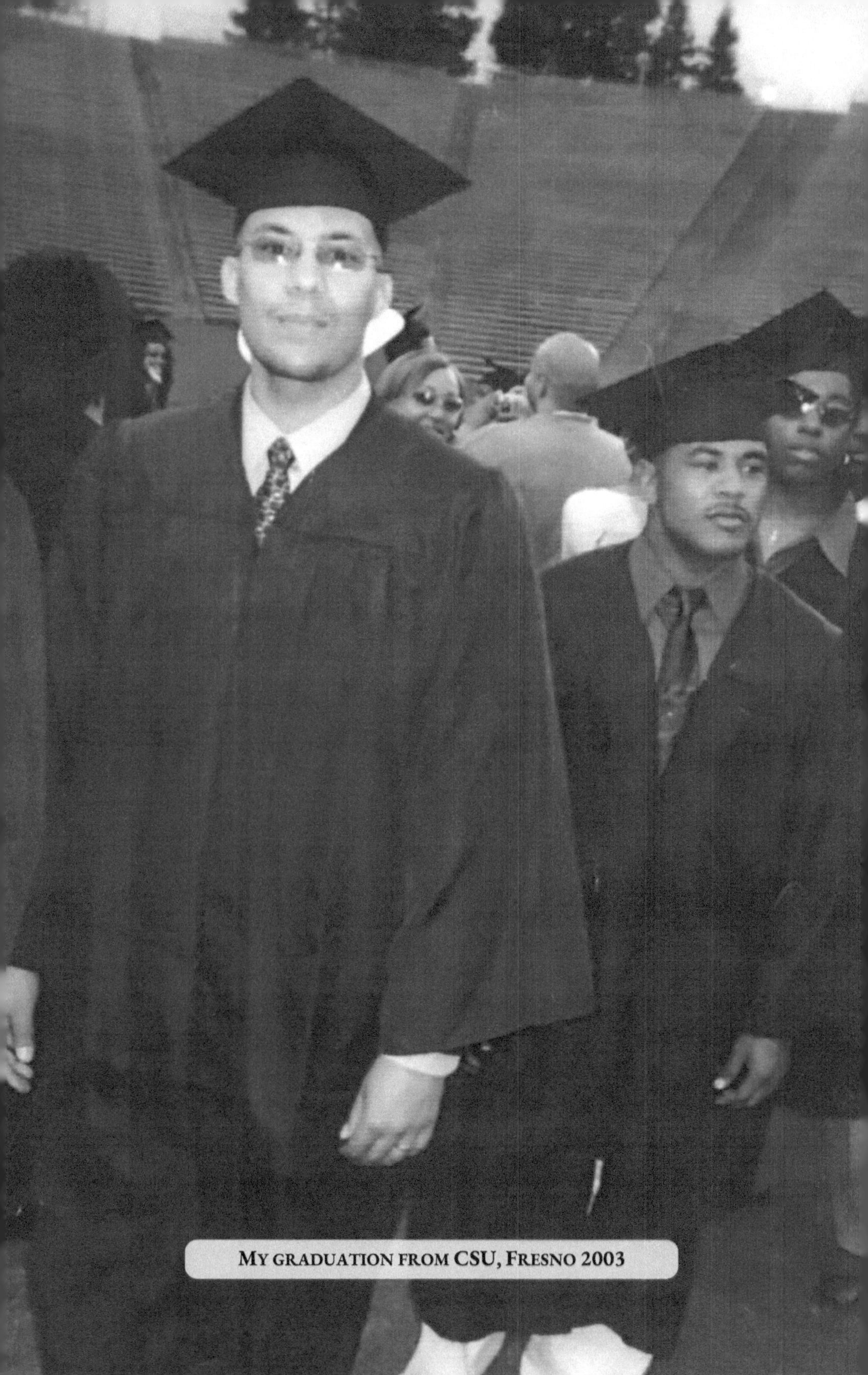

My graduation from CSU, Fresno 2003

CHAPTER 12

Mama's Gone

While I was in medical school at UCLA, there was a new curriculum that was pass/fail, but there was an opportunity to obtain a "letter of distinction" if you performed well enough on your exams. Obtaining this letter was the closest thing we had to demonstrating mastery of the material. I worked very hard, but also enjoyed the whole process. I was hitting my stride and had just finished my final exam, scoring high enough to earn a letter of distinction. I was excited to get home and celebrate with my family when I got a phone call from my aunt in Fresno: Mama had died.

When I was a child, Mama was my protector from all the negativity in the world. Her love saved me. She was the reason I never felt lost or alone back then. Even though she was not my biological mother, I was treated like her favorite child. She spoiled me to the extent that all of her children—my father, both uncles, and both aunts felt like I was, in some ways, their little brother. As a young child, I would ask Mama who her favorite child was, and she would tell me that I was. The very fact that I would ask such a question implied the degree to which I was spoiled. Although she spoiled me, she was God-fearing, and she instilled a set of strong morals which, later in my teenage years and young adulthood, kept me from doing something that could have led to my death or the death of others. Having hate in your heart can make any horrible thing possible. Having even a small portion of love deep in your heart can be enough to overcome the darkness of hate. Love produces a light that guides your path from the inside; it is like the inner voice that serves as your moral compass. Although I had much darkness around and in me, this light remained present even at my worst. I believe this kind of love is eternal and lives on beyond our lifespans. This love drives every decision we make that matters, and it convicts us when we do the wrong thing. I believe that to ignore this love is to ignore God. This gift of love that was passed on to me through my grandmother was a fulfillment of what the Bible calls the "Great Commission." Matthew 28:19 says that Jesus instructed the disciples to go out and make disciples of all nations. I can say without any doubt that God was introduced to me through Mama.

Mama had been hospitalized many times over the years for problems related to her heart failure. These episodes were often scary, but time after time, she would get better. Although the frequency of these episodes increased, the expectation that she would be home as usual became the norm, even with fear present. The inevitable and slow decline that is expected for someone with terminal cancer can sometimes be a bit more predictable because of the natural history of the disease. The episodic nature of heart disease can often lead to sudden death that strikes without warning. I was not prepared for Mama's death. Losing Mama to congestive heart failure was devastating. One of my driving influences in going into medicine was to become a cardiologist who could someday take care of her. Mama was everything to me growing up, and I felt like the cardiologists who cared for her over the years were the ones keeping her alive. The devastation from her loss led me to consider other career options as I approached my clinical years in medical school. In life, Mama was the first to introduce me to Christ, but in her death, she indirectly influenced my decision about how I would eventually spend my career serving others.

Driving back to Fresno for the funeral was very somber. I usually drove, but my wife could tell that I did not have the energy or focus to be safe behind the wheel. I gazed out the window as time and cars passed by. I was numb, and the flood of emotions was difficult to suppress, as I usually did. The kids were in the back seat, and I tried to subtly dab at the tears when one would escape, scratching the side of my eye while wiping with a tissue so that it was not obvious to them that I was crying. A deep and guttural whine snuck out when my wife noticed I was crying, and she placed her hand on my leg to console me. That touch was enough to prevent my pain from being trapped within my body. Even holding my breath was not enough to keep me from crying hysterically. I got it together and reverted to a few tears escaping as I stared out the passenger-side window. I apologized to the kids for crying, as they also quietly cried. They missed her very much as well. "It's okay, Dad." They were not used to seeing me cry, and this was likely the first time they had seen me in such a way.

The funeral was quite a blur. Many family members came from all over to pay their respects, and I do not recall many of them. Years later, some of those who attended would tell me that they were there, but I was in such a state of mind that I had zero recollection of any interaction with them. My mind could barely focus. Even maintaining the basics of eating and going to the bathroom required effort. I only remember sitting in the front of the funeral parlor on the left side of the room, right in front of the open casket. I did not like how Mama looked. They had put makeup on her, but not the way she wore it when she was alive. I stared at her hands, which still looked the way they did when she was alive. She had the same nail polish on that my Aunt Pat had put on for her before she died. Several times during the procession, I stood next to her and held her hand. The woman who raised me as her own was gone, and the thought of holding her hand for the last time brought back that guttural moan that I could not contain. Some came up to console me, but I have no idea who; my awareness of everything outside of my mind and Mama's hand was like the wind blowing past me. After the funeral, I had a few days to grieve before returning to medical school. I had completed my second year and was ready to move forward, knowing that was what Mama would have wanted. I prayed for strength to move forward despite my sadness and for God to lead me in the direction I was supposed to go. My desire to become a cardiologist had dissolved with Mama's death, so my sense of purpose was not as strong as it had been before.

I started my third year of medical school in surgery with every intention of getting it out of the way; I had no interest in the field. I had a preconceived notion that surgeons were largely mechanics for the body who received patients with problems already worked up and diagnosed by internists. My interest in medicine was based, in part, on enjoying the process of problem-solving. I wanted to be the one who figured out what was wrong with people. After starting the surgical clerkship, I discovered that there was a great deal of medicine and problem-solving involved in surgery.

On the first day of my general surgery rotation, I met my team, which consisted of a chief resident, a second-year resident, and an intern. When I met the second-year resident, he was in the intensive care unit (ICU) managing a patient. The patient was on a ventilator, medication to stabilize blood pressure, an insulin drip, multiple antibiotics, and nutritional support through a feeding tube. I asked him where the medical doctor was, and he looked at me as if I had insulted him. "What do you mean, medical doctor? I'm managing this patient. This is the surgical ICU." I had no idea there was such a thing as a surgical ICU. I quickly discovered that surgeons are trained not only to operate but also to manage complex medical problems in their surgical patients. The first two years of surgical residency place emphasis on medical management and critical care for surgical patients, while the last three years focus more on surgical skill development, team management, and leadership. Junior residents learn how to operate early in their training, but to be a safe doctor and surgeon, the trainee must be able to care for patients both inside and outside of the operating room.

While on my internal medicine rotation, I found myself longing to be back on the surgical service. Once I had determined that surgery would be my career choice, I needed to seek mentorship. I scheduled a meeting with the program director and had a shocking encounter. Surgeons tend to be busy and often straight to the point; this can sometimes be interpreted as rudeness, arrogance, or even cruelty, but what I experienced was a bit worse. When I arrived at the meeting, I was asked to come into his office and sit down. He was clearly busy and a bit distracted, looking through papers on his desk while asking me about my plans and interests. I shared with him that I wanted to pursue a career in academic surgery and that I was interested in going to a major academic center where I could get the best training. He looked bothered by this statement and suggested that I consider some smaller programs that would be easier to get into. He responded to my lack of response—and what was likely a look of disappointment on my face—with, "Well, how did you perform on your boards?" The "boards" refer to the United States Medical Licensing Examination (USMLE), which is taken in three parts. Step 1 of the boards is completed just before the clinical years of medical school. This exam, at that time, played a huge role in the decision-making process regarding which residency you get into. Some specialties are more competitive than others, and the best programs for each specialty will often give significant priority to those with high marks on this test. Thankfully, I worked very hard in medical school and achieved a score in the 99th percentile. I shared my score with this program director, and he had a look of complete shock that was quickly followed by a smirk. He said, "Well then, in that case, you can consider any program you want. You could stay here, go to Hopkins, Mass General, UCSF..." Then he paused and looked at me with his head tilted, as if bracing himself for bad news, and said, "But you don't have anything bad going on, right? Like a criminal record or anything like that?" I tried my best to hide my disgust. My inner monologue was screaming, *This racist sucker must be crazy*, but I kept my cool and smiled, stating, "No, sir, I am just like the other medical students here at UCLA; I have no criminal record." He said, "Well, you are going to be just fine." I left that encounter not only disappointed in what had just happened but knowing that I had no intention of staying there for my training.

Thankfully, the rest of my interactions with surgeons at UCLA were great. Various operations can be performed differently, and as you grow and develop as a surgeon, you carry those different methods with you and incorporate them into your practice. In the end, you become a reflection of the many who have trained you. Like the technical aspects of a case, there are personality traits and habits that you may also take with you. The chair of surgery was not only a technically fantastic surgeon who was fearless in the operating room (OR), but also one of the first people I think of regarding traits I adopted. He performed most of the liver transplants at UCLA, but also did complex liver resections for cancer. Like many surgeons, he would listen to music in the OR. One of the first questions he asked me in the OR was not about anatomy, but about his music. He asked me, "Do you know who this is?" I listened to all kinds of music and knew it was Al Green singing "Let's Stay Together." He was thrilled. "That's right! The Reverend Al Green!" he exclaimed with true excitement. To this day, I usually have music playing during every case, and I will often ask new students, residents, nurses, circulating nurses, surgical technicians, or even the anesthesiologist on the other side of the sterile drape if they know who the artist is or about some arbitrary fact related to the song.

The idea that we can be influenced in our personal lives and careers by the experiences we have with others was not a concept I had fully grasped until recently. Every individual has free will, which allows freedom of choice and expression, but either consciously or subconsciously, we are molded by these experiences. Awareness of this can sometimes aid in the process of self-improvement. Much of my fear as a child stemmed from the embarrassment I felt about what others thought of me due to my poverty and family members' drug use. I saw the differences between my life and those of my peers at school and sought money at an early age, by whatever means necessary, to hide who I was from others. I would spend the very little money we had on clothes similar to those of wealthier people. I would fight to keep my father in the house whenever he was high on crack so that the neighbors wouldn't think poorly of me. Sleepovers were allowed but rarely occurred because of the embarrassment caused by all the roaches in our house. It wasn't until I started to find friends in my neighborhood with the same problems that I began to let go of the belief that these things defined me. Knowing that I was not alone gave me the courage not to fear what others would think of me because of where I lived and the problems in my home. Through friendship with those who were like me, I learned to embrace and even make light of the things that once embarrassed me. This change in my outlook was also welcomed because I realized that I could help others who were like me by sharing my vulnerabilities. Years later, I came to understand that the very act of opening up was empowering because I no longer had anything to hide.

My path to discovering what I wanted to do with my life was, in many ways, a reflection of the process by which my experiences molded me. I liked the idea of being able to take control of a complex situation and possess a skill set that allowed me to manage a wide array of surgical problems. While we all need to ask for help from consultants for various problems, I wanted to be the one that others called for help. Feeling helpless was something I sought to escape as a young child. I wanted to have control; it is no coincidence that I decided to become a surgeon. Although my original plans to become a cardiologist were negatively influenced by Mama's death, she still had an impact on my career path. Mama was the light among the darkness in my life. She was my provider and protected me when I was vulnerable as a child. She was the first person to bring me to God and the most prominent influence in my choice to become a physician. Rest in peace, Gracie Mae Harris. Until my work is finished, I look forward to the day that we will be together again.

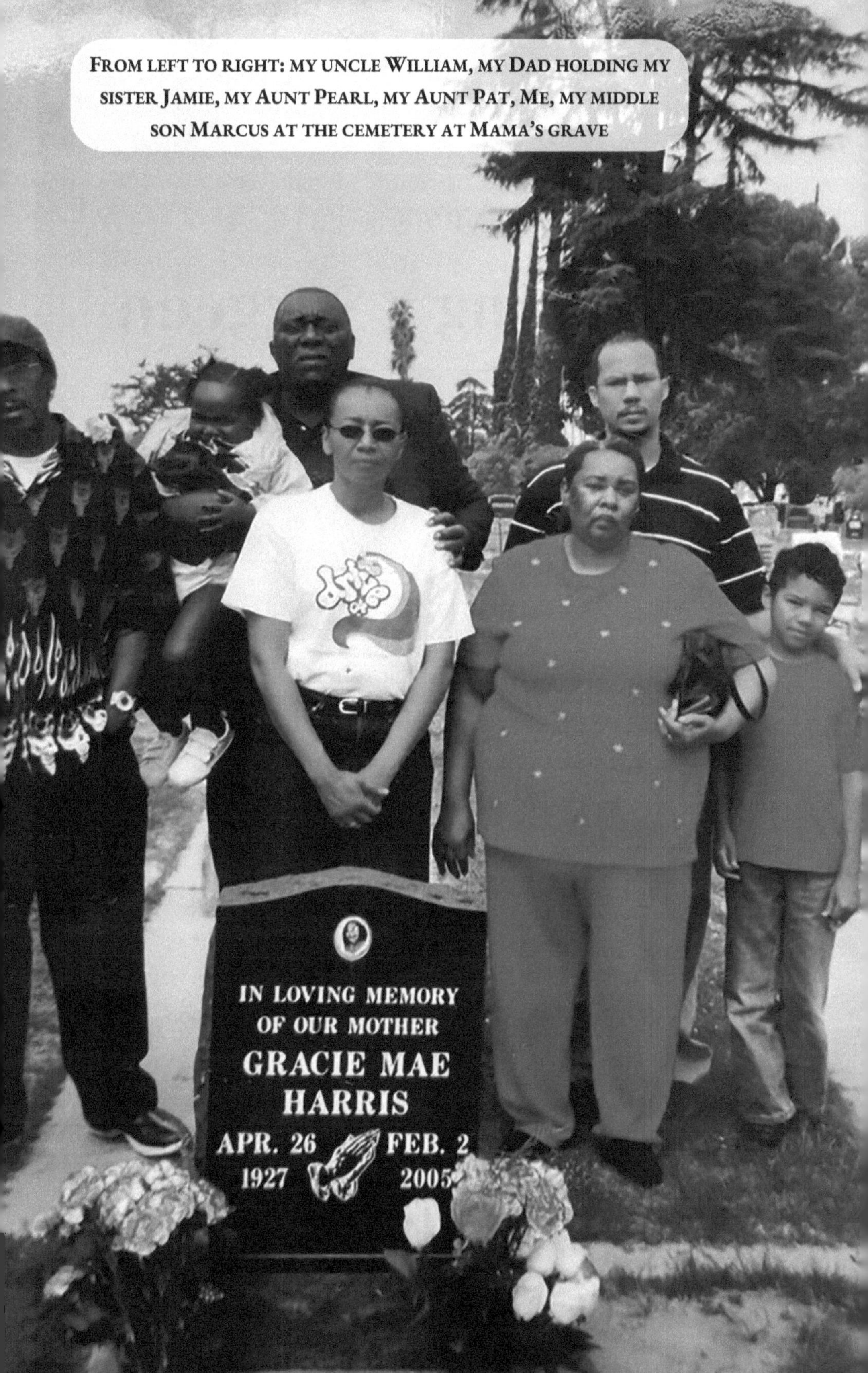

FROM LEFT TO RIGHT: MY UNCLE WILLIAM, MY DAD HOLDING MY SISTER JAMIE, MY AUNT PEARL, MY AUNT PAT, ME, MY MIDDLE SON MARCUS AT THE CEMETERY AT MAMA'S GRAVE

CHAPTER 13

Becoming a Surgeon

I could feel the darkness welcoming me as my eyes began to close. The warm heat from the vent felt so relaxing as I leaned on the steering wheel, trying not to fall asleep. My eyes snapped open as I realized I was not yet home in bed. I opened the window and let the cold winter air blast in. Despite the freezing wind and the knowledge that I was on the freeway going sixty miles per hour, my fatigue was so overwhelming that my eyes slowly started to close again. The darkness won again. The sudden drop of my head startled me awake just in time to see that I was headed straight for the wall of the freeway on the overpass at the curve, which happened to be more than 100 feet above the ground. That welcoming darkness was nearly the gateway to my eternal sleep. I had just completed a shift that was scheduled for 24 hours but lasted more than 30 hours because of several loose ends involving patient care that I could not ignore. I had no sleep and was constantly running from one patient to the next throughout the hospital.

My year as a surgical intern at Johns Hopkins Hospital was intense and a significant change from medical school. An intern is a new resident, fresh out of medical school. People often joke that the most dangerous time to be in an academic center is in July because that's when all the new interns start. At Johns Hopkins and many other academic centers, there is strong awareness of the need for increased supervision during this transition phase, so additional staff and senior residents are assigned to assist the new trainees. An 80-hour workweek restriction mandates that an intern or resident not spend more than 80 hours per week in the hospital. To the average American, 80 hours is the equivalent of two full-time jobs. But for residency, this was a significant improvement from what training had been like before the restrictions were established. As a resident, you are paid a modest salary while working an enormous number of hours. The restrictions do not take into account the many hours each week required to study for exams. Surgical residents have required readings and quizzes every week to prepare for a standardized exam each year. If your performance falls below a required threshold, you are in danger of being placed on academic probation. If you are unable to improve your academic performance, you are then at risk for remediation, where you may need to repeat the year or could even be terminated from the program. At the same time, every resident is evaluated multiple times during the academic year to make sure they are meeting all required milestones and performing at an appropriate level academically, technically, and professionally.

The 80-hour workweek, although mandatory, is difficult to regulate. Many institutions face the challenge of ensuring that residents log their hours accurately. I found it quite difficult to keep my work hours under 80 throughout my residency. Some who did not want to get in trouble always logged their hours as 79.5 when, in fact, they were sometimes working up to 120 hours a week. These residents were seen as dedicated and hardworking while remaining efficient on paper; I did not figure this out until late into my intern year. I logged all of my hours according to the time I spent in the hospital, and they often far exceeded the threshold. At times, no other provider was available to care for the patients who required certain services, so the responsibility fell to the residents and the attending physician. If the work was not completed, patients were not cared for. I would stay as long as it took to complete the majority of the work and then sign out smaller tasks to the intern on call that night. That intern, however, was always overwhelmed because they were covering up to five different services in one night. Expecting them to take care of all the unfinished work was unfair and unsafe for the patients.

Since a few others and I logged our hours accurately, we were labeled as inefficient and less capable than those who followed their duty-hour restrictions on paper but worked tirelessly without pay. Ignoring resident duty-hour violations can lead to the residency program being placed on probation by the governing body that monitors medical trainees. The intent is to protect the health and safety of residents, along with the patients under their care, by reducing medical errors due to sleep deprivation. Services that were once notorious for long hours became much more tolerable through the hiring of physician assistants and nurse practitioners. These ancillary staff members became invaluable members of the team and provided excellent care for our patients. By adding this additional resource to the team model, residents were allowed to spend more time in the operating room and less time staying late into the evening writing notes, discharge summaries, and completing other important tasks that did not necessarily add to the residents' education.

A surgical intern's main responsibility is to learn how to safely care for patients' medical problems. Interns are encouraged to go to the operating room as much as possible, but on many busy services, such as trauma and vascular surgery, the operative experience was lacking. Going from medical school to surgical residency is a significant transition; interns go from having very little responsibility as a student to caring for a high volume of patients under stressful circumstances, all while being sleep-deprived from being on call every third night of the week.

My first night on call was intimidating. I was so worried that I might harm a patient by making a mistake that when I was contacted by a nurse requesting an order for Tylenol, I had to look at the patient's entire history to make sure there was no medical reason I could not place the order. Did they have any liver disease? Were they taking any medications that could cross-react with Tylenol? Were they allergic to Tylenol? Why did they need this order? Did they have a planned procedure in which they were not supposed to have anything by mouth? You could spend forever looking for ways you might potentially harm a patient. The reality is that all of these things matter, but with experience, the mind is able to quickly answer all of these questions in a matter of seconds—if you know your patients.

As a surgical intern, I rotated on the plastic surgery service for several weeks. My first time on call was unforgettable, largely because of the trauma consult I was paged to evaluate. A middle-aged man with a scruffy beard was using a table saw in his garage and lost control of it.

Somehow, the saw bounced up and sliced through the side of his mouth, cutting all the way to the ear. The complex laceration was full thickness, from the skin to the inside of his mouth, and extended toward the bottom of his ear. The bleeding had already stopped by the time he arrived, but there was old blood clotted all around his face, mixed with some sort of black, tar-like material, which he said came from what he had cut through. I tried my best to maintain my composure while examining the patient, but in my head, I was freaking out. The injury to his face looked like something out of a horror movie. After completing my exam, I let him know I would step away for a moment to call my supervisor so we could make arrangements to take him to the operating room. The wound needed to be thoroughly cleaned and examined more extensively than I could perform in the emergency room.

I contacted my supervisor, who was a plastic surgery fellow, and told him about the patient. I explained in detail the extent of the injury and my concern for possible injury to his nerve and parotid duct. "Did he have paralysis on the left side?" he asked. I told him that the corner of his mouth was completely severed, so I wasn't going to ask him to smile to see if the nerve was cut, as that could potentially cause the wound to open up further and start bleeding again. He said, "Go back and clean off all the old blood and get a better exam. You should be able to close this laceration in the emergency room."

This was my first night on call for their service, and I was being asked to close up a patient's full-thickness facial laceration by myself in the emergency room. The Fellow told me what sutures to grab from the operating room for the different layers of the mouth and reassured me that I would be fine. I reluctantly went back to the patient after grabbing supplies and spoke with him about the plan. I obtained consent to wash out and repair his wound and began by cleaning off some of the black, sticky, tar-like material that was stuck to his bottom lip. As I wiped his lip with saline-moistened gauze, the blood that had clotted was brushed away, not only causing arterial bleeding but also revealing another laceration that had caused his entire bottom lip to detach from the middle and hang down. I held pressure on the bleeding vessel while trying to hide my terror. I grabbed suture material and carefully placed a stitch at the site of the bleeding vessel and tied it down to stop the bleeding. I told the patient that the laceration was a bit more extensive than I could repair safely at the bedside, so I would call my supervisor for assistance and likely take him to the operating room. I stepped away and called the Fellow back. "The man's lip is about to fall off! I need you to come in and help me!" I panicked.

He reluctantly came in and met me in the emergency room. After evaluating the patient, he agreed that this repair needed to be done in the operating room. He and the attending surgeon took the patient to the OR while I continued to see new consults.

Complications in surgery can often be avoided with safe practices, but if one thinks one can practice medicine without ever having complications, one is sadly mistaken. As a second-year surgery resident on the transplant service, I was asked to place a central line on a patient who was unable to have a peripheral IV placed because she had very small veins. I saw the patient, obtained consent for the procedure, and explained the reason for the procedure along with the risks and benefits. I gathered all the supplies and proceeded with the setup. I prepped and draped the patient with a nurse at the bedside to assist. We used a checklist as we performed our surgical time-out, a pause before starting to ensure we had consent, the correct patient, the correct planned procedure site, the correct patient position, all needed supplies, any medications necessary before the procedure, and that any safety concerns were addressed.

After completing the time-out, I used ultrasound to verify the location of the jugular vein on the right side of her neck and let the patient know she would feel a little sting from the needle stick, followed by a burning sensation from the numbing medication as I anesthetized the skin overlying the jugular vein. I then used the larger needle under ultrasound guidance to directly visualize and access the jugular vein, followed by the placement of a wire through the needle and into what I believed was the jugular vein. I removed the needle and made a small incision in the skin at the wire insertion site to allow enough room to then place the catheter into the vein over the wire. The catheter went in smoothly, and I removed the wire, but then there was pulsatile back-bleeding into the catheter with bright red blood. Venous blood is dark and non-pulsatile. There was no mistaking this; I had placed the catheter into the carotid artery. Fortunately, this was not one of the larger types of central lines we often place in trauma patients, so I removed the catheter and applied pressure for several minutes, hoping not to see a hematoma or external bleeding from the site.

The site looked good, without hematoma or bleeding, but I had to explain to the patient and my attending physician what had happened. The patient was very understanding, but I wasn't so sure that my attending would be. I not only failed at placing a central line, but also created a complication that now needed to be worked up. Sometimes the artery may lie just under the jugular vein, and even if you are watching with ultrasound, you may not realize you have gone through the vein and entered the artery beneath it. With experience, this type of problem happens less often, but I was not the most experienced at that time in my training. I called vascular surgery for advice, and they told me I should obtain a formal vascular ultrasound to ensure there was no injury to the artery that could require surgical intervention. I let the patient know the plan, ordered the study, and then went to my attending to share what had happened and what I planned to do. He listened to what I said and agreed with my plan. He then proceeded to tell me something I will never forget: "I see a number of residents in this position who have complications after a procedure. Some avoid taking responsibility and rely on their supervising residents to speak with the attending and the patient. This can become a habit that creates mistrust between the patient and the doctor. Facing your mistakes the way you did and taking responsibility to do what you can to help, without running away from the problem, will help you later in your career. Some doctors avoid the patient after they have made a mistake. Never do this, because if you do, you will lose that patient's trust."

The patient did not require surgery related to this complication, but the lesson learned still had a significant impact. Taking responsibility for my patient meant doing so regardless of the outcome or the time of day. Their life was being entrusted to my care, and I had a duty to perform to the best of my ability to achieve the best possible outcome. If the mark is not hit, we do not simply give up and pass this responsibility to another. When we take this ride with our patients, we stay on board for both the good and the bad. Complications cannot be eliminated completely; there are variables we cannot predict or control. What we *can* do is learn from our mistakes and the mistakes of others in order to become better. We can also learn to identify when the risks of a procedure significantly outweigh the potential benefits. Some operations are elective and may not need to be done in the immediate future, or at all. Having a conversation with the patient should lead to a better understanding of the expected outcome and all the possible risks. If the risks of forgoing the procedure could lead to a poor outcome, the patient may be more inclined to move forward with surgery, but they need to know what to expect during recovery. Even simple considerations, such as expected pain levels, potential for bruising and swelling, activity limitations, the possibility of recurrence, and other routine aspects of the operation, can aid the patient's decision-making.

Learning how to care for surgical patients requires a broad knowledge base of both medicine and surgery. Being a surgeon involves more than what is done in the operating room. To achieve good outcomes, a surgeon must first consider the patient as a whole, not only the disease. A stereotype exists, and unfortunately holds true for some surgeons, who are seen as "hammers" viewing each patient's surgical problem as a "nail." Patients are individuals with complex medical, emotional, social, and spiritual circumstances that we must be willing to consider before we act. If we neglect any of these aspects, it could lead to a poor outcome despite performing a technically sound operation. For acute care surgery, these considerations can sometimes be minimized due to the urgent nature of the surgical problem, but this can sometimes make them even more important because the stakes are much higher and the time available to consider these factors is short for both the surgeon and the patient. It may seem like an easy decision to rush to the OR if someone has a life-threatening surgical disease, but if they cannot speak for themselves due to their illness and have a living will that states they have certain restrictions on what they would want done in such a situation, this must be respected. If the patient has a family member who wants to go against the patient's wishes in order to save their life, we can only do so if the patient decides to suspend their previously stated wishes. Learning how to navigate when *not* to operate is sometimes more difficult than simply taking the patient to the OR because of all the other variables that must be considered in providing what is considered the optimal outcome for the patient.

CHAPTER 14

The Sinister Side

Historically, being different or outside the norm has often been challenging. Even something as simple as left-handedness has been viewed negatively. Many medical terms derive from Latin, and the term *sinister*, now associated with evil or threat, originated from the Latin word *sinistra*, meaning left. To this day, ophthalmology and optometry refer to the left eye as *oculus sinister*. It is estimated that approximately 10 percent of the world's population is left-handed, and only one percent exhibits mixed handedness. In surgery, instruments are predominantly designed for the right hand, forcing left-handed individuals to either become proficient with their right hand, adapt to using right-handed instruments with their left, or develop proficiency in both. Although left-handed instruments exist, requesting them as a resident could mean requiring an entire extra set, risking a mix-up and causing confusion during procedures. For me, adapting to using my non-dominant hand was difficult. As an intern, I stubbornly believed it was illogical to abandon my natural hand. I wrote and ate with my left hand, so why not operate with it? The problem was that every surgeon who trained me was right-handed, and every case was set up for a right-handed surgeon using right-handed instruments. Even the surgeon's position relative to the patient influences the operation.

Initially, I operated with my left hand, but I soon realized that the surgeons training me were confused and, at times, frustrated because they had to rethink their approach. A stitch thrown by a right-handed surgeon from the patient's right side is typically forehanded, but the same stitch from a left-handed surgeon would be reversed from that position. Switching sides with the attending surgeon seemed natural, but most were uncomfortable with that. Surgeons are creatures of habit, and as Dr. John Cameron, the former Johns Hopkins Chair of Surgery, famously said, "Do the same thing, the same way, every time." To my knowledge, no resident ever dared ask Dr. Cameron to switch sides in the operating room. Such a request was unthinkable. Adaptation was the resident's responsibility, not the attending's.

My first real understanding of the frustration of operating as a left-handed surgeon with a right-handed attending occurred during my trauma service internship. The attending on call was in the OR with the chief resident when a patient arrived in the emergency room with a gunshot wound to the abdomen. With no other resident available, our Head of Trauma, Dr. Efron, the backup attending, took the patient to the OR. He needed an assistant, and upon seeing me enter, he immediately appeared disappointed to have been assigned an intern.

"You have got to be kidding me," he muttered, shaking his head. "You had better get ready for a beating because this is not an intern-level case." I don't recall my response, but with the chief resident tied up, Dr. Efron was stuck with me. I scrubbed in, bracing myself for the inevitable.

The patient had a small bowel injury requiring resection and anastomosis. A bowel anastomosis can be performed using staples or hand sewing. While stapling is faster and easier, many Johns Hopkins-trained surgeons, following the tradition of the first Chair of Surgery, Dr. Halsted, were trained in hand-sewn anastomoses. Although hand sewing remains a valuable skill, most surgeons prefer stapled anastomoses for their speed and ease. Consequently, many surgeons today lack sufficient experience with hand sewing to master the technique. If they encounter a situation requiring it, they may face technical difficulties, potentially leading to leaks. Dr. Efron typically trained his residents, including me, using the hand-sewn method to prepare us for independent practice. As we prepared to sew the bowel together, Dr. Efron grew frustrated when I began to stitch with my left hand. Again, he exclaimed, "You have got to be kidding me!" He stared at me as if I were some perplexing equation. Despite his disappointment in operating with an intern, especially a left-handed one with no experience in hand-sewn bowel anastomoses, he guided me through the procedure. It was a painful experience for both of us. He allowed me to operate with my left hand but constantly complained about having to do everything backward. I completed the case, but every stitch was met with criticism. I was unaware of the intricacies involved in creating this connection. Stitches that are too wide or too shallow can lead to life-threatening leaks. Stitches that are too deep can catch the posterior wall and occlude the anastomosis. An insufficient diameter can cause an obstruction. Failure to close the space between blood supplies can allow another loop of bowel to slip in, kink, and cause a blockage. The intense teaching during that case taught me more about the importance of surgical technique than any previous experience.

I left the OR disappointed in myself but determined to improve. Still unwilling to switch to operating with my right hand, I practiced relentlessly with my left. I carried a right-handed needle driver in my left hand between patient rounds, practicing palming the instrument while opening and closing it smoothly. Over time, I became skilled with my left hand, but this didn't alleviate the concerns of the right-handed surgeons training me because they still had to adjust the case setup. I learned to throw a stitch left-handed from the patient's right side by angling my body, but this encroached on the attending's personal space to the left of the patient. Some didn't mind, but most seemed displeased even if the work was done correctly. After only a few instances during my intern year, I realized I was missing valuable training when right-handed attendings—and they were *all* right-handed—performed critical steps themselves despite my capabilities.

I learned to perform most basic cases left-handed, and during laparoscopic procedures, my handedness was less apparent because everyone focused on the video monitor rather than my hands. Switching hands laparoscopically was easier, possibly due to my childhood video game experience. Gradually, I began using my right hand more and more, eventually matching the style of the surgeon I was working with.

By my third year, I was using my right hand effortlessly for most cases. After hundreds of cases, I had become ambidextrous.

Before my rotations began, an old-school surgeon contacted me, saying he'd heard I was left-handed and that I would be operating with my right hand on his service. Had I not already transitioned, I likely would have been offended and anxious about the rotation. Instead of revealing my transition, I simply agreed, allowing him to believe I was still operating left-handed. I doubt any right-handed surgeon has been instructed to stop using their dominant hand. I agreed to use my non-dominant hand for the entire month without complaint, but during my second rotation with him, I decided to demonstrate the benefit of using my left hand when appropriate. Sometimes, the natural hand for placing a stitch might require an awkward opposite-direction throw, but switching hands can be a much easier alternative. This old-school surgeon had a revelation and, for the first time, recognized the advantage of being able to throw a stitch with either hand. To this day, I use the hand best suited for the task. My surgical training forced me to become ambidextrous, and although challenging at times, it made me a better surgeon.

As an academic surgeon, I teach during every operation. I am committed to resident education because sharing my knowledge with future surgeons has an exponential benefit. By explaining and demonstrating the what, how, and why, I can help not only the patient at hand but also future patients who may benefit from what I taught their surgeon. When I operate with left-handed surgeons, I recognize some of the struggles I once faced, but I can adapt and help them optimize their body positioning to complete each task.

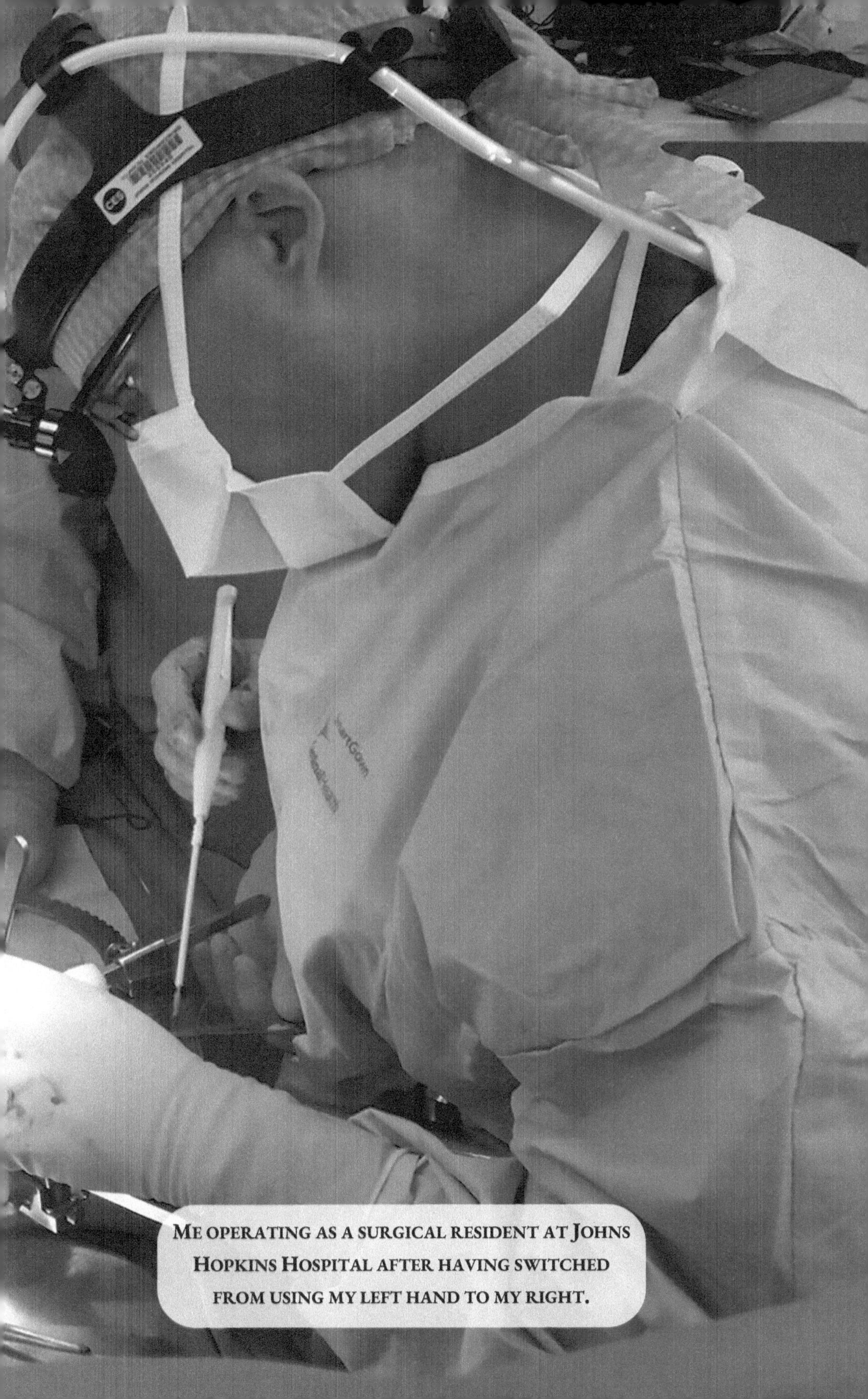

ME OPERATING AS A SURGICAL RESIDENT AT JOHNS HOPKINS HOSPITAL AFTER HAVING SWITCHED FROM USING MY LEFT HAND TO MY RIGHT.

I openly share my strategy for accommodating the surgeons who trained me, but regardless of a resident's dominant hand preference, the most important thing is to prioritize what is needed to best care for their patients. The attending physician who complains won't be there when the resident becomes the attending, so even though we all want to make a good impression and avoid complaints, the resident's individual needs must be considered when determining what is best for them. Countless individual variables must be considered for every surgeon.

Our trainees deserve the necessary support to become the best surgeons they can be. Achieving proficiency and practice readiness sometimes requires extra effort from both the resident and the attending. This obligation extends beyond the individual patient, encompassing all future patients under the trainee's care. To be a successful academic surgeon, we must consistently provide excellent patient care while preparing our residents to become excellent, independent surgeons, regardless of their handedness.

CHAPTER 15

Blood in the Water

Surgical training is so intense that it can lead some of the most brilliant and technically skilled residents to abandon their course of study altogether. While this is frowned upon by the surgical community, it is often more courageous, and a better alternative, to leave the program in search of a better career path than to stick it out in a profession you no longer want to pursue. The dropout rate for surgical residency has decreased significantly over the years, largely due to the 80-hour workweek, but also because of a growing cultural shift. Still, a proportion of surgeons at every institution believe their residents should be treated with the same degree of toughness with which they were trained.

When a resident is perceived as lacking confidence, usually due to being soft-spoken and respectful, they can become an easy target for verbal abuse by their supervising residents and attending surgeons. In my surgical intern class, we had a great colleague who was intelligent and hardworking but socially a bit reserved. One fellow resident witnessed the surgical hazing he endured while on the same service and said it was like he was surrounded by sharks with blood in the water. The attending would harshly criticize him about a clinical decision he made, and a supervising resident would then ridicule him further. It seemed like every time he reported his treatment plans, there was a look of exasperation as they listened, followed by them tearing his plan apart. This treatment continued for most of his intern year, and he ultimately decided to leave the program to pursue a different career path in anesthesiology. A few years later, a very similar situation occurred with another resident who left the program after the second year to pursue training in emergency medicine instead.

Leaving a training program in order to pursue other interests is far better than going into the field and potentially spending the majority of one's life being miserable. I believe this happens more often than we realize. These physicians are more likely to suffer burnout, which may lead to depression, disconnection from their patients, substance abuse, or even suicidal ideation. While these problems can occur in any field, I witnessed one such incident during my first few years of residency. An anesthesia resident was found abusing drugs he obtained from the operating room. He was brought to the emergency room one day after overdosing and was found unconscious with a bottle of propofol falling out of his pocket. Propofol is the same drug that contributed to the death of Michael Jackson. It is a safe drug when used for its intended purpose—inducing anesthesia—but if self-administered or given to another by someone not qualified to care for patients for this purpose, it can be very dangerous. Propofol causes loss of consciousness and can simultaneously produce respiratory arrest and a drop in blood pressure, which can ultimately lead to death. Fortunately, this anesthesia resident was revived and placed into mandatory rehabilitation, which helped him overcome his addiction. He was able to return to his residency after rehabilitation and successfully complete the program.

Physician burnout and depression have led some physicians to feel that there is no way out other than taking their own lives. According to the American Foundation for Suicide Prevention, physicians have a higher rate of suicide than the general population, with men being almost one-and-a-half times more likely and women more than two times more likely to die by suicide. During my residency at Johns Hopkins, we did have one resident who attempted suicide. They survived, and for confidentiality reasons, I will not disclose any specifics about this individual or their circumstances, but I will share how it made me feel. All residents work long hours together, and like a family, we had good times and bad times. In a high-stress work environment, we can sometimes be short or even abrasive with one another. At times, I was not very kind to some of those I worked with. When this resident attempted suicide, I hadn't been on service with them for a few months. I kept thinking back, trying to remember if there was ever a moment when I had said anything that could have contributed to their depression and subsequent decision to end their life. Thankfully, I never recalled any problems with this resident, but in a field like surgery, where some of us are so focused on patient care, we often neglect the emotional needs of those around us. Over the years, I have made a conscious effort to be more aware of and respectful toward others' feelings because I never know what they may be going through.

Surgical training can sometimes feel like pruning; cutting the branches of a plant at certain critical points may seem painful, but it promotes growth. "You've got 45 minutes." That was what the surgical intensivist (a physician who specializes in the care of critically ill patients) said when I woke her up to tell her that the patient I was caring for in her surgical ICU wasn't doing very well. Most intensivists work one-week shifts in the ICU and leave after evening rounds, but not this one. She would sleep in the unit so that if there were any problems, she was there to do everything she could to take care of the patient. She had very high standards regarding patient care and expected no less from her trainees. Looking back on this time with her, I appreciate how it helped me develop into the surgeon I am today. While going through it, I cannot say it was a pleasurable experience. There was an expectation to know everything about your patients and at the same time, be able to manage their needs while in the ICU: how to appropriately identify and manage every type of shock; how and when to perform invasive procedures; how to manage complex medications, including calculating the appropriate dose for aminoglycosides (a potentially toxic antibiotic sometimes required for multidrug-resistant bacteria); how to calculate the nutritional requirements for a specific patient's needs; how to write orders for the correct IV or enteral nutrition; how to adjust ventilator settings, including when to choose the correct mode; and any other aspect surrounding the care of ICU patients.

At two that morning, my patient was still in shock after a long case in the OR, despite my giving her multiple fluid boluses and starting medication to support her blood pressure. I knew I had to place a central line and potentially a Swan-Ganz catheter (a pulmonary artery catheter used for advanced hemodynamic monitoring and medication delivery) to help manage her fluid resuscitation. But first, I had to wake up my program director. After explaining what was going on with the patient and my plan, she agreed and said, "You've got 45 minutes." That was how long she expected me to take to place a large central line, called a Cordis catheter, and the Swan-Ganz catheter. I was expected to check the patient's baseline cardiac output using the Swan-Ganz catheter and then administer a fluid bolus to determine whether cardiac output improved with the additional volume. This whole process typically should not take more than 45 minutes under optimal circumstances, but on this early morning, conditions were far from optimal.

To place the central line, we used ultrasound guidance to visualize the internal jugular vein and insert the catheter under direct vision over a wire in a process referred to as the Seldinger technique. This was my first problem: someone had borrowed the ultrasound and forgotten to return it to the ICU. I had to spend the first fifteen minutes looking for the ultrasound. I then had to gather my supplies and finally began the process of placing the line thirty minutes later. It was around this time that my program director decided to check on how things were going. She was not aware that I had spent the last thirty minutes locating the ultrasound and assembling supplies, so she was livid that I had not already placed the line. As I was prepping the patient, she walked into the room and asked, "Why isn't that line in yet?" I started to explain, but she did not want to hear any excuses. Her focus was on the patient and ensuring I was doing what she believed should have already been done. I remained silent, stayed calm, and focused on the task while under her watchful eye. I told myself this was a test to see whether I could perform under duress. As I was setting up for the procedure, I made sure not to show any fear through my demeanor or in my hands. Developing a tremor because of anxiety or fear while performing procedures is not a favorable quality for a surgeon. During stressful times like this, I still remind myself that God has brought me through so many hurdles in life, so why start freaking out now? I placed the line without difficulty, and we were able to keep the patient alive and well.

Trauma is a significant part of surgical training at Johns Hopkins. Since the hospital is located in inner-city Baltimore, operative trauma cases from victims of violent crimes are common. Despite our location, our patient population at Hopkins is very diverse. One day you can be caring for a drug dealer who was shot multiple times, and the next, you may be operating on royalty who traveled from the other side of the world to have their pancreatic cancer treated at Hopkins. We were taught to provide excellent care to all, regardless of the patient's walk of life.

When patients who have been shot or stabbed lose vital signs en route to the hospital or in the ER, many require an emergency room thoracotomy. This procedure involves using a scalpel to open the chest on the left side, cutting through the skin, subcutaneous fat, and muscle to gain immediate access to the heart, lung, and aorta. By placing a vascular clamp on the aorta, arterial bleeding in the abdomen can be controlled in a manner similar to shutting off the main water line if you have a burst pipe in your home. The sac around the heart, the pericardium, is opened, and if an injury is found, it can be repaired. Once access to the heart is gained, cardiac massage can be performed to manually pump it if it has stopped beating.

Over my years of training at Johns Hopkins, I cared for hundreds of gunshot and stabbing victims who required surgical intervention, some requiring thoracotomy for cardiac injuries. Many, unfortunately, were beyond help on arrival, having lost vital signs too long beforehand to be resuscitated, but some of those who arrived before becoming brain dead were successfully resuscitated. There was rarely a reason to perform a thoracotomy on a patient with blunt, non-penetrating injuries, but one day, while on call at one of our satellite hospitals, I was paged to the emergency room for a middle-aged man who had been in a severe car accident and was en route. He had been partly ejected through the driver's-side window when his vehicle rolled over and landed on his chest. He was crushed by the weight of the vehicle and was extricated by paramedics and firefighters on the scene.

Upon arrival, the man had labored breathing that was shallow and rapid. With each inhaled breath, his chest moved inward rather than expanding, exhibiting paradoxical chest movement consistent with multiple rib fractures on both sides. The man was barely able to speak due to the severity of his injuries, but he was still conscious and had vital signs. He was in shock with a rapid heart rate, low blood pressure, and cool extremities. For any trauma patient, we follow a management algorithm of ABCs: Airway, Breathing, and Circulation. The patient's ability to maintain and protect his airway was compromised, so we had to place a breathing tube. We then checked for breath sounds, and they were diminished and distant on both sides. Given the flail chest (where three or more ribs are broken in two or more places), his hemodynamic instability, and decreased breath sounds, we immediately placed bilateral chest tubes for bilateral pneumothoraces (collapsed lungs). This slightly improved his heart rate and blood pressure. We placed two large-bore intravenous lines and started giving IV fluids, followed by blood. At the same time, we performed a Focused Assessment with Sonography for Trauma (FAST) at the bedside, an ultrasound of the abdomen and heart used to detect blood in the abdomen or around the heart. We found blood in both areas, consistent with intra-abdominal hemorrhage and injury to the heart.

So much blood surrounded the heart that we were concerned about cardiac tamponade, a condition in which the fluid or blood around the heart creates such pressure within the pericardial sac that the heart cannot adequately fill. When the heart cannot properly fill, it cannot pump blood to the body. This condition leads to shock and eventually death if it is not treated. This is an unusual presentation for blunt trauma. Usually, cardiac tamponade is caused by penetrating trauma directly to the heart, but there was no external sign of penetration to the chest. Cardiac tamponade can occur in some patients with certain viral infections or chronic medical conditions in which fluid builds up in this space, but in this setting, our suspicion for such causes was low. We were concerned that his flail chest was the cause. One of his broken ribs could have penetrated not only his lungs, causing bilateral pneumothoraces, but also the heart.

We called the operating room to prepare for our arrival and then called the on-call surgery attending physician to drive in from home so we could take the patient to the OR for emergent surgical exploration.

The surgical attending would take more than 45 minutes to get to the hospital—time we did not have to spare. We had to get the patient to the OR immediately to begin without him. We rushed the patient into the OR and prepared his chest and abdomen with a sterile cleaning solution. We placed a sterile drape on the patient as he was connected to the ventilator and anesthesia was administered by the anesthesiologist. The patient was hypotensive at this time, with his systolic blood pressure in the 60s and a heart rate above 160 beats per minute, so the anesthesia attending, who had experience with cardiac anesthesia, decided to place a specialized ultrasound probe into the esophagus to visualize the heart from the inside of the chest. The attending confirmed that there was severe cardiac tamponade. We performed a median sternotomy by making an incision directly over the sternum and using a sternal saw to divide the sternum in half, gaining direct access to the heart. We found that the pericardium was bulging and tense, without a clear site of penetration by a rib, contrary to our initial expectation. We opened the pericardium and found blood within the pericardial sac, as we suspected. After releasing the blood, the patient's blood pressure improved immediately, and his heart rate came down to a near-normal level.

We then examined the beating heart, looking for the source of the bleeding, and found that part of the right atrium, called the right atrial appendage, had ruptured. This part of the heart is not as thick as the tougher ventricles. When the vehicle landed on the man's chest, his heart ruptured at its weakest, most vulnerable area. The hole was only a few millimeters in diameter, and it took a single suture to close the defect. Just then, our attending walked into the OR. We updated him, and he joined the case to help us finish the operation. After closing the chest, we moved on to the abdomen to identify the source of bleeding there and found liver lacerations. We were able to gain control of the bleeding by placing multiple large sutures to close the laceration after placing specialized hemostatic absorbable material into the laceration. We explored the rest of the abdomen and found no further injuries. We closed the abdomen and escorted the patient to the surgical ICU.

We spoke to the family, his wife and adult child, who were in the waiting area. They were not with him at the time of the accident and were terrified. We shared the extent of his injuries and what we did to treat them. I could see relief wash over their faces. They had heard of the severity of the accident and appeared to have been bracing themselves to hear that he had not survived. The patient had a challenging recovery, requiring an additional ten days in the hospital, three of them in the ICU, but he did survive and walk out of the hospital. He returned to the clinic for his follow-up appointments looking great. He returned to work and moved on with his life. Although these circumstances are rare, and many do not make it to the hospital in time to be saved, it is often cases like this, which a surgeon may encounter only once in a lifetime, that inspire him or her to remain in the field. The opportunity and honor to help people in this way serve as the fuel to endure all the sleepless nights on call, waiting for the next person who may need his or her help.

CHAPTER 16

My Father's Last Call

I was on the trauma surgery service, named after the first chair of surgery at Johns Hopkins, Halsted. This service was responsible for every trauma that came to Johns Hopkins, along with the vast majority of urgent and emergent surgeries. I was on call as a senior on the service and had just received sign-out from the overnight resident, who was post-call. Shortly after receiving the pager, it went off. The notification read, "MVC, ETA 10 minutes." Many of our traumas were classified as either penetrating (gunshot wounds, stabbings) or non-penetrating (car accidents, falls). Penetrating traumas often required emergency surgery, while non-penetrating traumas were usually non-operative for our team unless severe. Blunt injuries could lead to emergency surgical needs, but a large portion were related to head and bone injuries, so we often relied on neurosurgery and orthopedic surgery for these cases. I do not recall the details of this particular MVC beyond it being non-operative for our service, largely because of the call that I received shortly after evaluating the patient and confirming that they were stable.

I had just walked out of the trauma bay into the small hallway that led to the computed tomography (CT) scanner. Trauma suites, by design, have rapid access to CT scans due to the urgent need for rapid diagnosis in a closely monitored setting. As I walked into the back hallway toward the CT room, my cell phone rang. I saw that it was my wife on the caller ID and became uneasy because it was rare for her to call me while I was on service, knowing that I was often fully occupied with patient care. I answered, and she told me, "They're coding your dad right now."

Despite some of his shortcomings, my father was the first man who had a significant influence in my life. Both positive and negative influences can result in building character; my father contributed his share of both. As the product of an affair that my grandmother had with another man, my dad looked different from his two older brothers and, consequently, was treated differently. My grandmother returned to her alcoholic husband while pregnant with my father. They had two more children together, my two aunts, but my father was never treated like the others. My father didn't learn the truth about his biological father until he was a teenager. When he was 12, he was left in Arizona with his grandmother while his mother (Mama) moved to California with her new boyfriend and two youngest kids. Her new boyfriend was abusive and also a drunk. My father began living on his own as a teenager, earning money from doing yard work and other odd jobs. After earning enough money to buy a car, he drove to California in search of his mother.

The new boyfriend was not only abusive and a drunk, but he was also a child molester who sexually abused my oldest aunt throughout her childhood. Many of these things were hidden from the family, as they often are by victims, because of embarrassment and fear. Once my aunt revealed the abuse, my grandmother confronted her boyfriend with the accusations, only to be severely beaten. My uncle caught wind of the incident and took justice into his own hands by shooting him in the stomach. He survived, but out of fear of going to jail, he did not report that it was my uncle who shot him.

My father returned to stay with my grandmother after her boyfriend was shot. Like my grandmother, he never graduated from middle school because of his circumstances and subsequently never furthered his education. My father had dyslexia and had great difficulty with reading and writing. His math skills were adequate to above average for everyday business. He spoke using big words that were often used in the wrong context, but he was quite charismatic, with a genius-level street IQ. His laugh and his energy were contagious. He was able to earn an income through hustling. He never had a formal nine-to-five job, but he was always working different angles to make a dollar. As he became a young adult, he had enough money to live in a nice neighborhood and purchased several nice classic cars.

Shortly after my father met my biological mother, they moved into a two-story home where they stayed until she left him several months later. My father provided my mother with material possessions but was jealous and had a temper. My father was an entrepreneur of the ghetto. He worked with the ladies of the night as a pimp, and he also dealt in illegal pharmaceuticals before he himself became a victim of the industry. He and my mother eventually began using the drugs which my father sold. The saying "don't get high on your own supply" was perhaps not well known at the time. Their finances began to suffer. The drugs increased my father's innate jealousy and paranoia. He never trusted banks while he was in his specialized line of work, so he kept large amounts of money in the home. One day, after my grandmother had put me down for a nap, two masked men with guns broke into the house and tied my grandmother up, demanding money and drugs. My grandmother knew that my dad kept a large sum of money under a gigantic Mexican sombrero that was in his room, but she didn't reveal this to them. The perpetrators ransacked the house, completely missing the loot under the sombrero. After only finding some jewelry and other valuables, they stormed out, leaving my grandmother tied up and me in my crib.

Several months after this incident, my biological mother left my father and asked my grandmother to take care of me. My father did not raise me, but he was often around. I was raised believing that my grandmother was my mother. My father was unable to get off drugs and leave the lifestyle he was living, so my grandmother took full custody of me and became my legal guardian. It took my father several years to distance himself from the drug life. He was always somewhat paranoid, but crack took this pre-existing personality dysfunction to a whole different level of instability. Even though he wanted to take custody of me, he was hardly fit to care for himself at that time.

At six feet three inches and more than 300 pounds, my dad was quite intimidating, especially when he was high. My dad had a dark complexion with big, round eyes. His bright white teeth and the small gap between his two front teeth stood out in contrast to his dark skin tone. He resembled a cross between the late comedian Bernie Mac and the reggae artist Shabba Ranks. His dress was often unpredictable. At times, he wore a suit and tie with leather shoes that were purchased at the Salvation Army, as he refused to pay full price for new clothes. At other times, he could be found in ragged, oil-stained jeans and some random tropical shirt topped with a captain's sailor hat. When I was around five years old, he bought matching sailor hats for both of us to wear while riding around in his 1937 pearl-white convertible Jaguar with suicide doors. My dad loved his classic cars, and before he got hooked on crack, he always had a few fancy vintage cars around. He also loved jewelry. The fingers on each hand were often adorned with multiple gold rings, and multiple gold chains with various pendants hung from his neck.

My dad used jewelry as a source of income when times were tough for him, but outside of the crack years, he always found a way to get the jewelry back from the pawnshop. For the three to four years that he was using drugs, he could not keep any valuable possessions and lost everything to the point of homelessness. During that time, he lived in front of our house on the southeast side of Fresno in a small, broken-down RV. All of his money was spent on crack, and despite the embarrassment of having him live in our front yard, I would often sneak food out to him. Toward the end of his drug era, Mama would not let him come into the house because of all the trouble he brought. Even though I was ashamed of the way he acted when he was on drugs, I was glad that he was close by, where I knew he was safe. Before he had the

RV, he would disappear for weeks and sometimes months at a time, and I would not know if he was safe or even alive.

Unlike my uncle and aunt, who would use drugs in the bathroom next to my room and then go to their room or somewhere else to enjoy their temporary high, my dad turned into a confused and paranoid monster. He would leave the bathroom with eyes wide, sweat beading down his dark face, and lips curled with a look of terror on his face. When on crack, he appeared as if he were being told there was a bomb that could go off at any moment and that if he stepped in the wrong place, bumped into a piece of furniture, or told anyone what the problem was, the bomb would explode. He erratically stared in all directions as droplets poured down his face, and his hands patted his shirt and pants pockets as though he had forgotten his keys or his crack pipe in the bathroom. All the while, his eyes and face shifted from the ground to the wall and even up to the ceiling.

I stared at him, afraid that he would go outside and top his last chaotic scene by stripping nude or smoking crack in the front yard. He never streaked or smoked out front, but he always made a scene. He would walk out into the front yard near the sidewalk and pace back and forth, with that ever-present sweat and his hands searching for whatever he thought he'd lost. This would go on for several minutes until the peak of the crack high began to fade and he felt comfortable enough to then retreat to the inside of his rundown RV.

Fortunately, my dad had already cleaned up his life by the time I met my wife. I was always thankful that my wife only got to know my father after he was clean. She moved in with me when she was 16 years old and pregnant with our first son. She did see other family members of mine while they were still hooked on drugs, largely crack and heroin, and it tarnished her image of them. She was never raised around drugs, so this type of behavior was quite foreign to her. Her father did have a drinking problem, but he was never violent. Most of my family members who struggled with drugs managed to isolate themselves from everyone else while they were high, but not my father. Crack cocaine intensified his preexisting paranoia. It was not until I made it to medical school that I was able to figure out what was wrong with my dad. During my study of psychiatric disorders, I used people I knew personally, along with characters from movies or television, as examples of the many different types of mental illnesses to help memorize the information for the test.

After my dad stopped using drugs, he lived in a small home on the west side of Fresno and even started a non-profit organization called "For All People There Is Hope." Through this non-profit organization, my dad collected food from grocery stores and restaurants that was near expiration and delivered it to homeless shelters and families in need around the city. Since my wife never knew my father during the crack years of his life, she never lost respect for him the way she did for some of my other family members who were still hooked on drugs when we first met. To this day, Rosina still has difficulty getting along with some of my surviving family members who were hooked on crack back then. She saw the lowest points of what the drug did to them and the lack of care and respect they showed for themselves and their families while in pursuit of drugs. We could be down to our last bottle of formula, with barely enough money to buy more, and still be pressured into "lending" money to them. We quickly learned never to lend money to a crackhead because repayment was unlikely, and requests for more money often continued.

Much later in life, my dad decided to start another family with a woman younger than me who, unfortunately, struggled with drug addiction. He believed he could help her become sober, but this was unsuccessful. They had two children together but were unable to make the relationship work. My father took custody of the first child, my half-sister, who was born while her mother was in prison. My father wanted to have a mother figure for my half-sister, so he tried to reconcile the relationship after the woman's release from prison. They were on-and-off for a few years, but she continued to struggle with drugs. They eventually had another child together, my half-brother. She initially retained custody of him while my father kept my half-sister. He worried often about my brother's safety because she remained involved with drugs and did not have a stable home for him. At her lowest point, she was living in a homeless tent community with my brother when he was around four years old. She was caught up in drugs and prostitution at that time, so my father took custody of my brother as well.

My dad struggled greatly while trying to take care of my half-siblings by himself. My brother had spent his early childhood in an unsafe environment on the streets, where he was exposed to drugs and prostitution. He had a number of behavioral issues. My sister did not get along well with my brother, so their relationship further complicated matters. Despite my father's limited parenting skills, his lack of a partner to help, and the challenging circumstances with the children, he somehow managed to provide for them and keep them in school. My father enrolled my brother in sports as a way to channel his energy and anger in a productive direction. My brother struggled in school, but having an outlet through sports seemed to help keep him motivated academically.

My father had struggled academically as a child because of dyslexia and reading difficulties that persisted into adulthood. Although he was sometimes hard on my brother, he understood the challenges he faced because he saw himself in my brother.

During one Thanksgiving, my wife, our three children, and I went to my grandmother's house for dinner with my father and his two youngest children. As we sat down and waited for dinner, my dad casually mentioned, "I ran into your brother, Calvin, the other day." Perplexed, I asked, "Who is Calvin?" My dad responded, "You know, your brother Calvin . . . Remember the time I took you to the park to play with the remote-control boats with that little boy? That was your brother." I had no response to this absurdity.

I was aware of an older sibling whom I had met once a few years earlier. He was a Crip in Los Angeles and serving time in prison. My father told me about this mysterious brother when I was a teenager and showed me a few stereotypical-looking prison photos of him posing in a crouched position while mean-mugging the camera. I had no serious motivation to connect with this mysterious brother, although he did stay with my father for a short period after his release from prison, where I met him for the first and only time. This was the first time I had heard about any half-brother named Calvin. I vaguely recalled going to the park to play with remote-control boats and running into a mother with her child whom my dad talked to, but at no time did he mention that this random kid was my brother.

He then nonchalantly dropped a second surprise, saying, "You know, your sister Rochelle lives just down the street." Halfway through a swallow of turkey with stuffing, I almost choked at this revelation. I had had enough. There were apparently half-siblings, some of whom I have never met to this day, who were living in the same city and even down the street from me. At first, I laughed and took this as a joke, but he was dead serious. During the times he was not present throughout my childhood, he had apparently been busy elsewhere. I never investigated. It was a bit much for me to process. Having been raised by my grandmother, with my father not always around, I imagined that he must have lived this other life while he was away. He was quite the player. I recalled the many times my father would go to great lengths to flirt with complete strangers at the store, waiting at bus stops, or at the DMV. After getting clean from drugs, it seemed as though his addictive personality persisted, shifting its focus toward relationships with women.

My dad never had the responsibility of raising children on his own until he had my little sister and brother. Despite having had multiple children before this, he was quite new to the whole parenting gig. After I moved across the country for my surgical residency at Johns Hopkins, he would often call me seeking advice on how to get the kids to behave. He was quite stressed, and I would advise him as if they were my own misbehaving children. We often rewarded good behavior with positive reinforcement and withheld privileges when they did not meet expected goals, tasks, or behaviors. While this strategy worked well for us, we raised our children from birth and had their entire lives to help shape them. My father did have my sister shortly after her birth, since her mother was in prison, but he didn't have the support of a spouse to help him. With regard to my brother, he was not brought into the home until after he had been exposed to drugs, homelessness, and prostitution during the early years of his childhood. The strategies that worked for my children did not work for these kids, especially not for my brother. I didn't fully understand the difficulty of raising these kids until after my dad's passing, when I brought them into our home and tried to take over their care.

My father was a big man, and although he was tall, he was significantly overweight. He often said he wanted to eliminate sugar from his diet but never truly broke the habit. I have fond and humorous memories of him cutting and eating about one-third of an entire cake for himself. It was funny at the time, but looking back, I now realize he had challenges with self-control that shifted from drugs to food. This dependence on unhealthy eating habits did not serve him well and contributed to chronic high blood pressure, which ultimately led to his death. My father was not very trusting of doctors and often felt he was being used or taken advantage of. Although my father had somewhat mystical patterns of thinking, which I suspect may have reflected a schizotypal personality disorder, I did believe some of his concerns were valid.

When doctors don't explain why they are prescribing a medication or describe what to expect, patients are less likely to continue taking the medication. Hypertension is often asymptomatic, so treatment adherence can be low if the importance of controlling it is not clearly understood. My father was usually prescribed three different medications for high blood pressure, but because of his trust issues and lack of symptoms, he often stopped taking his medication whenever he didn't feel well.

My father believed the government had listening devices everywhere and that his ideas were being taken and used before he could implement them. This delusion controlled his life and made him paranoid. I often tried to use logic, even as a young child, to explain why these ideas were unlikely, but there was no convincing my father otherwise. Mental illness was not unfamiliar to me. I was not only raised around my father and other family members who were on drugs, but I also had an aunt with schizophrenia who heard voices and had delusions of her own, which she expressed openly. My aunt firmly believed that the famous basketball player, Michael Jordan, communicated with her through speakers in the wall. Like my father, logic did not work with her. What she heard in her mind was her reality, and there was no persuading her otherwise. Between the crackheads and the unusual statements made by my aunt, I was very selective about who I brought home as a child.

When my father called me one late evening to tell me he had awoken with severe chest pain, he said, "I felt like that was it." His seven- and ten-year-old children were with him at the time. The kids were picked up by their mother, who had separated from my father a couple of years earlier. I told him he needed to call an ambulance and go to the emergency room immediately. He had long-standing hypertension and was often noncompliant with his medications. I called the hospital and spoke with his nurse to find out how he was doing. She informed me that he was stable but was still having pain despite being given pain medication and nitroglycerin. He had an electrocardiogram (ECG) and laboratory tests that showed no signs of a heart attack. I trusted that they were evaluating him appropriately to determine what may have been causing the pain, so I didn't speak to the doctor to investigate further. What I didn't know was that the pain was radiating to his back, and there was no plan in place to rule out a tear in the wall of the aorta—an acute aortic dissection. If a CT scan had been done, the diagnosis might have been made, and an emergency cardiac surgery consultation for repair might have saved him.

My father was admitted to a monitored bed for atypical angina (heart-related chest pain) and went into cardiac arrest the following morning when the tear in his aorta ruptured into the space around his left lung and into the sac around his heart. I was on call that day for the trauma service at Johns Hopkins and was just finishing up with a patient when I received the call from my wife that his heart had stopped and they were actively performing CPR on him. I called the section chief for trauma, Dr. David Efron, who was very supportive and made all necessary arrangements to cover my shift and worked with our program director, Dr. Pam Lipsett, to ensure that I could leave that day to be with my father. Little did I know that both of these leaders in my department would also serve as some of my family's greatest supporters just 19 months later when tragedy would once again strike our family.

As I was leaving the hospital, my wife updated me that they were unable to resuscitate my father, and he had passed away. I flew back to California that day, arriving in the early evening. I headed straight to the hospital where he had died. A hospital representative and a security guard escorted me to the morgue where his body had been placed. They opened one of the metal doors to reveal a metal gurney holding my father's body inside a white plastic bag. They pulled the gurney out just about halfway and then walked out of the room, saying they would give me time with my father. I could see the outline of his head through the bag, and I stared at the zipper for a few minutes before reaching for it. I placed my hand on my father's head from outside the plastic bag and felt the cold firmness beneath. I began to pray for strength as tears started to spill over and flow. I imagined that his face would be one of pain and agony. I unzipped the bag and was surprised to find that he looked very peaceful; it almost seemed as though he had a faint grin. My tears continued as I touched my father's forehead, and I immediately felt that there was a deeper meaning to that moment. My father spent many of his last years struggling as a single dad trying to care for my half-brother and half-sister, but now he was at peace. Their mother was not able to take care of them adequately, so I felt that this was my father's way of telling me that it was meant for me to take over their care. I would later discover the depth of my father's struggles in raising them after going through a difficult custody battle for guardianship with their mother.

Before navigating the legal system to seek custody of the kids, I had to figure out how to bury my father. My father had no life insurance policy, apart from a small one my grandmother had paid for many years earlier, which covered only half of the funeral costs. My father had no savings account, and the only things of value were a few old cars and some scrap metal, which I had to sell to cover the remaining burial expenses. The funeral was emotionally draining and reminiscent of the pain I felt when we buried Mama almost seven years earlier, to the day. My grandmother and father both died in the same month I was born.

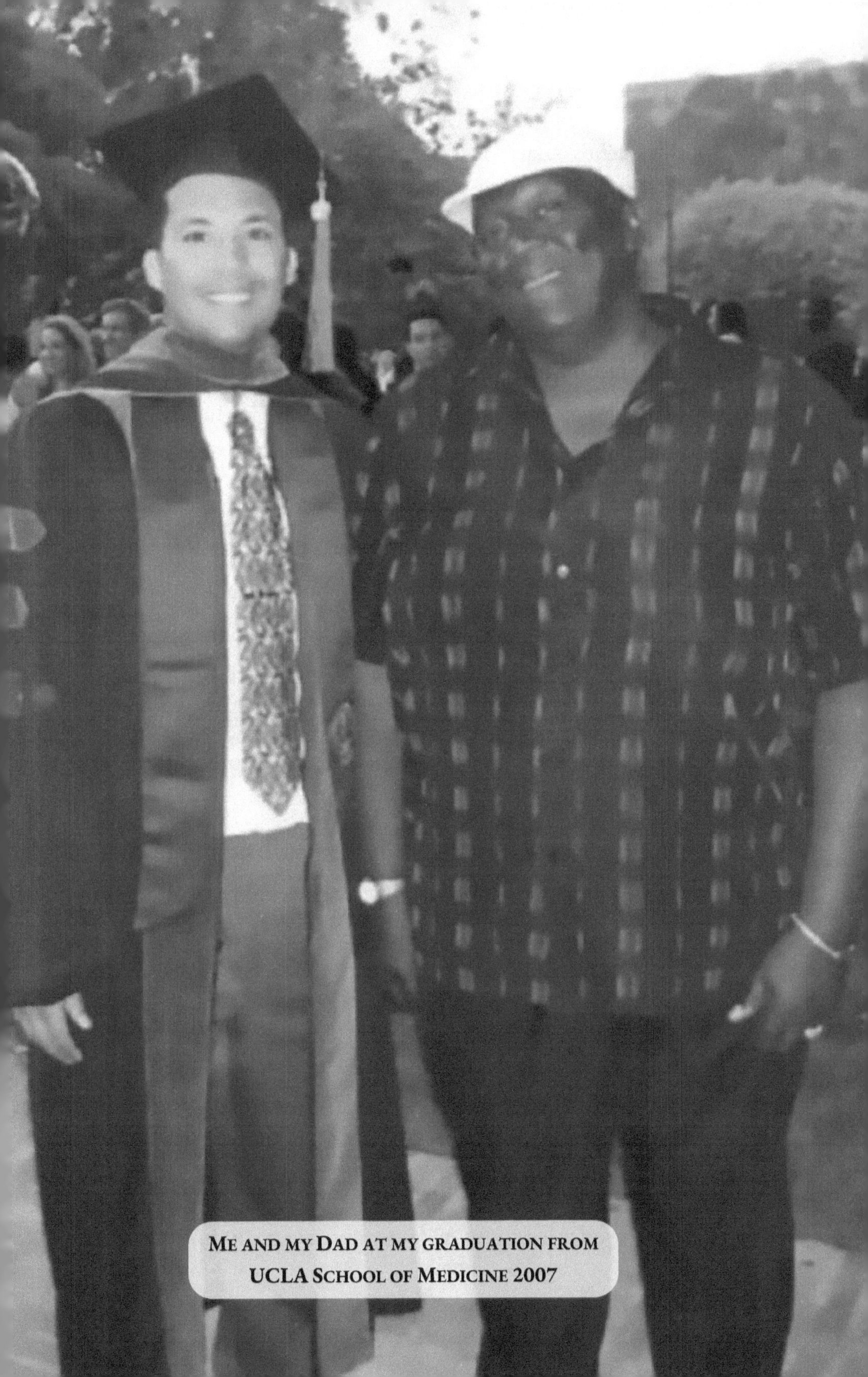

ME AND MY DAD AT MY GRADUATION FROM
UCLA SCHOOL OF MEDICINE 2007

On a resident's salary, I could not afford all the expenses that became necessary. Thankfully, my Johns Hopkins family donated money to help us with travel costs, and we were able to hire a lawyer to assist in the guardianship process for the kids.

The kids were staying with their mother in a small apartment in a rough area of Fresno when we obtained custody a few months later and brought them to Maryland. It was not until we brought them home that I began to understand the challenges my father had faced.

We enrolled them in the same school as my daughter, who was one grade level above my sister. The first week was chaotic as we adjusted to the logistics of caring for two additional kids, but we made it work. The problems arose as their behavioral issues became more severe. My brother started getting into fights with the other kids at school, and after a few weeks of multiple meetings with teachers and learning he had taken a knife from home to class, we knew we needed to seek professional help for him.

He began having severe tantrums, during which he became violent and inconsolable without an obvious trigger. He would throw all of the toys and clothes we had bought for him out of the room whenever he became upset and would thrash violently if anyone attempted to interact with him during these episodes. My sister, however, did quite well in school and seemed very motivated to succeed. She was highly competitive, which can be a positive trait, but this created frequent conflict with my daughter and wife. On multiple occasions, my sister would "play fight" with my daughter, who would end up getting hurt. One of these episodes led to my wife getting caught up in the middle, refereeing a dispute, while I took a passive role and stayed out of the situation. I was not as supportive as I should have been, and my wife became upset and went outside for a walk.

As she left, my sister smiled at her mischievously, wiggled her fingers in a teasing way, and said, "Byyyyeeeeeeeee." These kids were slowly tearing us apart, and I was beginning to realize how naïve I had been to believe we could use the same parenting strategies with them that we had used with our own children.

Overwhelmed financially and emotionally, we hit the final breaking point about one year into the kids' time with us. We had made many trips to the pawnshop and sold nearly every possession of value we had, except for our wedding rings, which we contemplated pawning on at least one occasion.

We had been forced to file for bankruptcy the year before due to the overwhelming debt we had accrued over the years, but it was not the financial burden that ultimately led us to accept that we were not equipped to continue caring for my siblings any longer. It was the inability to change their behaviors, which were affecting our family and slowly pushing us apart.

Every morning before I leave for work, my routine is to gently kiss my wife on the cheek. She rarely wakes up, and if she does, I give her a proper kiss before leaving. Because of my brother's violent behavior and his history of taking knives from the kitchen cabinet, my wife feared that she might one day be stabbed in her sleep. One morning, as I was about to leave, I gave my wife the routine peck on the cheek, and she woke up startled, with a look of terror in her eyes, afraid she was about to be attacked. This persistent feeling of fear, and the sense that we were no longer safe in our own home, led to the difficult decision to return my siblings to California. Their mother was deemed unfit to take care of them, so they both had to enter foster care where they remained for a couple of years before their mother passed away.

Years later, after completing my surgical residency at Johns Hopkins, I struggled to understand the meaning behind all of this. I tried to figure out where I had gone wrong. For many years, I felt guilty for my inability to take care of them. When I saw the look of peace on my father's face after I opened the body bag, I interpreted it as a sign that he had passed away believing I would take care of his children. I have since come to terms with the fact that we did our best, and although we had them for only a year, we were able to remove them from the volatile environment they had been living in. My sister, Jamie, has grown into a very charismatic woman who is a strong advocate for individuals who have gone through the foster care system. She has continued the work through my father's non-profit, "For All People There Is Hope," and she frequently participates in motivational speaking engagements to raise awareness about challenges within the foster care system.

My brother had a more difficult transition into his teenage years. He had frequent fights with other kids in the foster homes where he was raised and moved from one home to another without any stability. He ended up being incarcerated as a minor and continued along this path into adulthood, where he remains at the time of writing for committing crimes similar to those my father was involved in as a young adult.

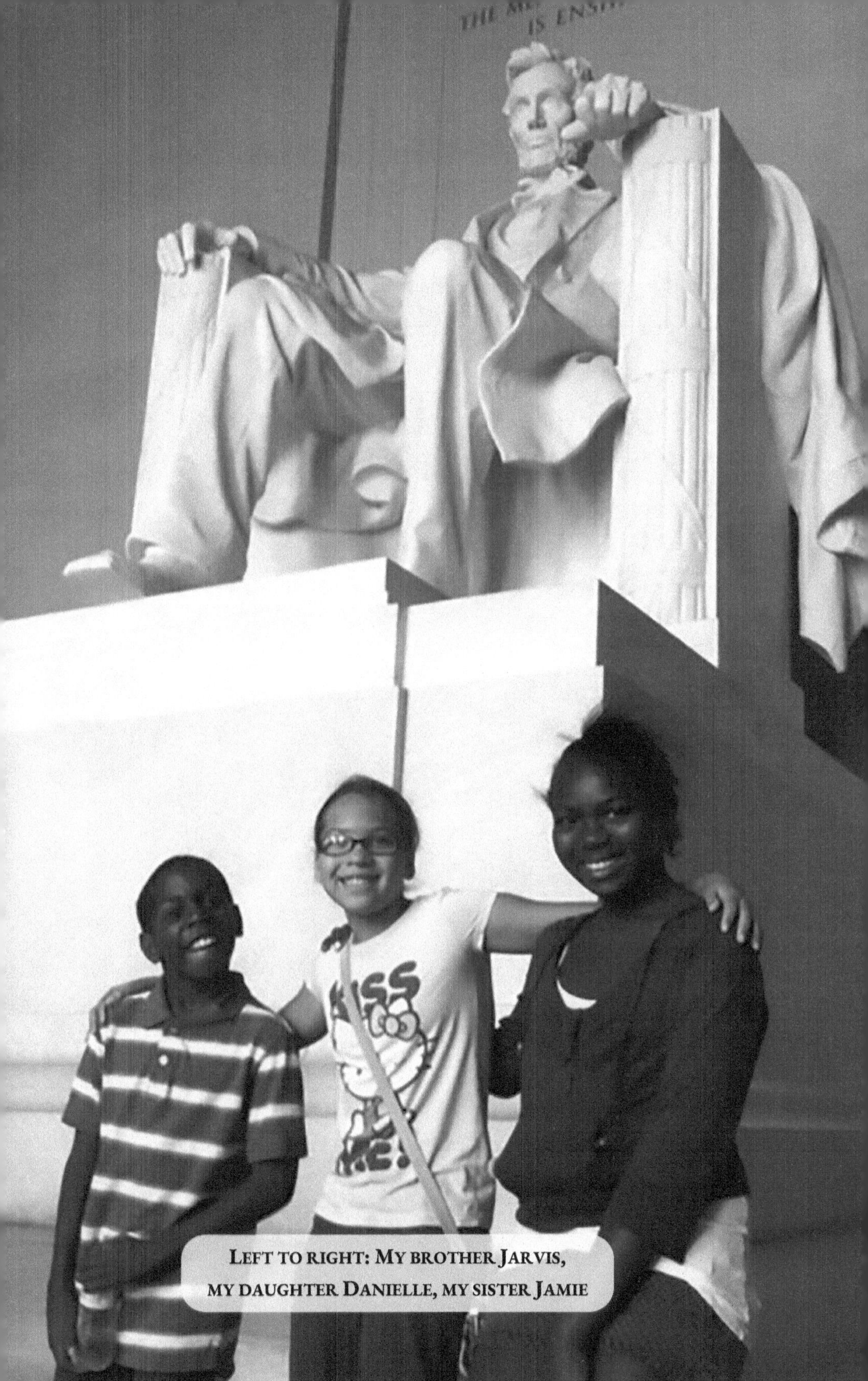

Left to right: My brother Jarvis, my daughter Danielle, my sister Jamie

I have slowly accepted that we did our best under the circumstances involving my siblings and have entrusted that worry and guilt to the Lord. My family was not equipped to take on the additional responsibility of raising two more children at that time, and our decision to try was not a mistake, but we underestimated the challenges we would face. If we had been at a different phase in our lives, perhaps things would have worked out differently. My past failures do not haunt me; they serve as lessons that help me make better decisions moving forward.

CHAPTER 17

Rwanda

One of the big attractions for me in ranking Johns Hopkins as my number-one choice for residency was not only its reputation for producing talented and successful leaders in the field, but also its international experience. Traditionally, all Hopkins surgical trainees were expected to travel internationally for six months during their fourth year of training. The program covered the cost of the resident's travel and expenses, as well as those of his or her spouse and children. Unfortunately, because of increasing case volume requirements in the United States, the program had to cut the international rotation down to one month and make it optional.

I jumped at the opportunity to spend a month in Rwanda, where I worked on the acute care surgery service with a retired thoracic surgeon from the United States. Our responsibility was to supervise the surgical interns on the service Monday through Friday, and on the weekends, we explored the country. I stayed in an apartment that was right around the corner from the public hospital in the city of Kigali. The country is quite beautiful but has a very recent dark past, with its version of a modern-day Holocaust not so long ago.

Two major tribes of people occupied the country: the Hutu and the Tutsi. On April 6, 1994, a plane carrying the Rwandan president, Habyarimana, was shot down. He was a member of the Hutu tribe. It is not known who shot the plane down with a surface-to-air missile, killing the president and all who were aboard, but this sparked roadblocks by Hutu extremists throughout the country. These extremists began executing all members of the Tutsi tribe, along with any Hutus who did not join in the efforts. According to the BBC, an estimated 800,000 people were murdered in only 100 days. There had been smaller-scale attempts during prior civil wars over the years, in which the Hutus had attempted to kill the Tutsi, but this Rwandan genocide shocked the world after the truth came out. What was happening at the time was not called a genocide but a civil war. The United Nations (UN) had troops in the country, but they did not intervene. After several Belgians were killed, the UN withdrew from the country, leaving hundreds of thousands to be murdered.

Books and movies depict the events surrounding the Rwandan genocide. The famous movie starring Don Cheadle, *Hotel Rwanda*, was one of many such stories that highlight some of the tragedies that took place there. This hotel, Hôtel des Mille Collines, was only a little over a mile away from my apartment, so I used the gym there multiple times during my stay. More than 1,200 Tutsis and Hutu moderates found refuge there during the genocide and were saved. Everywhere else in the country, including churches, stadiums, UN headquarters, and the very hospital where I worked every day, was unable to protect those who sought sanctuary. Don Cheadle's character was the hotel manager, Paul Rusesabagina, a Hutu who had married a Tutsi. He was able to save his wife by hiding her with their children in the hotel, but her parents were murdered in the genocide. Using the resources of the hotel, he bribed the Hutu militia with alcohol and other lavish gifts, which were otherwise used for the hotel's high-profile guests. The gym where I worked out was right next to the hotel bar and the swimming pool that served as the water supply for the refugees after the water was shut off.

I toured many of the sites the killers invaded. I visited two churches that had been memorialized by preserving them in their post-genocide condition. Hundreds of bones from the bodies were stacked on display in a small makeshift mausoleum in the back of one church, alongside countless piles of clothes and personal belongings of the victims on the floor. There were even baby clothes, bottles, shoes, and other such items from infants who were also indiscriminately murdered there. One skeleton was left in the basement of the church, preserved intact, to highlight how barbaric the killers were. The body was that of a woman who was brutally tortured and killed with a spear shoved through her body from her anus to her mouth. Her skeleton was placed in a glass coffin for visitors to see. As you walk through the church and look up at the ceiling, you can see sunlight shining through the bullet holes from where the militia climbed onto the roof and shot down into the church. An overwhelming feeling of sadness permeated everywhere I looked.

Through brainwashing propaganda broadcast over the radio, reminiscent of Nazi Germany, the Hutu militia were able to dehumanize the Tutsi to strengthen their commitment to their cause.

The history of hostility between the two tribes originated when Rwanda was colonized by Germany in the 1890s, followed by the Belgians in 1916, who ruled until after World War II. The Belgians supported the Tutsi minority over the Hutu majority, giving them political power. This led to further animosity and, eventually, revolts. Members of the Hutu and Tutsi tribes were eventually mandated to carry identification cards indicating their tribal affiliation. For those of mixed tribal background, the dominant inheritance was paternal. During the genocide, if the father was Hutu and the mother Tutsi, the individual could survive only if they agreed to assist in the murder of all Tutsi, including their own Tutsi mothers and wives. Hutus who tried to protect Tutsi or did not assist in the genocidal efforts were also killed.

Throughout Rwanda, from April 7 to July 15, 1994, innocent Tutsi men, women, and children were slaughtered. Hutus who refused to participate were also killed. Bodies were in the streets, in ditches, throughout stores, and in homes. Even the hospital where I worked each day was a site of genocide, where Tutsi patients and employees were identified and dragged out to be executed. Eventually, the Tutsi who escaped to Uganda were able to rebuild the Rwandan army, with support from Uganda's military, and end the genocide. Many of the Hutu militia escaped to neighboring countries, primarily the Democratic Republic of the Congo, but many were captured and held responsible for their war crimes.

When I arrived in Rwanda just over fifteen years after the genocide, much had improved, but the aftermath of the tragedy was still palpable. In advance of my arrival, besides the necessary vaccinations and paperwork requesting hospital privileges, I was also instructed on various cultural considerations. Tribal classification was no longer used, and it was taboo to ask citizens which tribe they belonged to. To eliminate division, all Rwandans were considered equal. Although peaceful for the most part, occasional terrorist attacks still took place along the western Congo–Rwanda border. While many perpetrators were apprehended for their crimes, the number of people who actively participated in the genocide was so vast that not all could be taken into custody. Rumors circulated that some who played minor roles in the genocide served time in jail for their crimes and later worked at the hospital.

Like other hospitals around the world, the hospital's surgical program had morbidity and mortality meetings, along with daily sign-out to the surgical staff each morning regarding new patients admitted overnight. The residency program was relatively new and had a bare-bones surgical staff for attending coverage, so they relied heavily on their international colleagues from the United States who rotated through for supervision and teaching. After hearing the daily updates from the interns each morning, including complications and deaths that occurred almost daily, it became obvious that the interns were performing the cases at night by themselves.

In the United States, at smaller hospitals where I rotated, there were some instances in which the attending physician was not in-house and we had to take the patient to the OR immediately to save the patient's life.

Such examples have become rare due to requirements for trauma surgeons to be in the hospital while on call, but in Rwanda, it was frowned upon for interns to call for help. During each morning report, the interns would discuss the patients on whom they'd operated overnight, state the presentation, the operation performed, and the postoperative status. After hearing about a number of deaths from overnight operations that I felt were due to technical errors, I decided to take call overnight on the days when there was no senior coverage so I could supervise and assist the interns who were having trouble. We would often operate most of the night, covering all urgent and emergent surgical cases.

The surgical experience was similar to that in the United States, with common problems like appendicitis, cholecystitis, which is inflammation of the gallbladder, bowel obstructions, and trauma. There were also diseases that were quite unique and rarely seen in the United States, such as abdominal tuberculosis and other infectious diseases. Antibiotics weren't readily available for all patients who needed them, so some people survived the operation but subsequently died from sepsis due to lack of sufficient medical treatment. Families sometimes had to purchase and bring in dressing supplies from home because of the limited supply of materials. Those who did not have family to provide assistance, nor the personal finances to pay for their medication or dressings, had to go without. The hospital was free of charge with respect to services rendered, but the materials and medications, which were often donated, were hard to come by.

The trauma experience was not quite as intense as what we see in Baltimore, but there were a few machete attacks and one man with multiple gunshot wounds from an assault rifle on whom we operated. The man was shot while trying to smuggle drugs across the border and had injuries to the small bowel and colon. Our suture supply was significantly depleted, but thankfully we had enough to repair all of his injuries, and he survived. Many of our traumas were from motor scooter–related injuries. Throughout the city, motor scooters served as affordable taxis; it was common practice for Rwandans to quickly travel from one place to another around the city by riding these dangerous machines. Before seeing some of the horrible injuries that resulted from this practice, I, too, used this resource to travel to different sites and was terrified on a few occasions as we zipped between cars in the city and almost crashed into pedestrians or other vehicles.

After each case in the operating room, we would go to the ER to see the next surgical consult. The ER was so overcrowded that people lined the walls and sat or even lay on the floor, waiting to be evaluated. One of the first trauma patients I cared for was a young woman who was brought in from the street after being struck by a bus. She was placed on a stretcher, where her most obvious problem was the significant hemorrhage and deformity of her right leg. The more alarming issue was that she was lying still, taking very shallow breaths, and moving very little air. While most were distracted by the severe leg injury and surrounded her mangled limb, I had the intern place a tourniquet above the area of the bleeding while I focused on the ABCs of trauma (airway, breathing, and circulation). She did not respond to my verbal commands, did not open her eyes, and only withdrew slightly with sternal rub. She was not safely protecting her airway, so we placed a breathing tube and started ventilating her using a handheld Ambu bag. I listened to breath sounds, which were equal, thereby ruling out any significant pneumothorax. I felt her pulse, which was weak, so we placed two large-bore intravenous lines and gave her IV fluids while wheeling her to the operating room.

The leg injuries were too extensive for repair. She required an above-the-knee amputation to control the blood loss. The case was uneventful, and she survived to leave the hospital, but it was easy to see how, if the fundamentals of trauma resuscitation (ABCs) had been neglected for much longer, the woman likely would have died or suffered an anoxic brain injury.

The operating theaters were basic, with limited supplies. Suture material was of high value, and there were no gastrointestinal stapling devices to perform bowel resections or anastomoses, so all procedures had to be performed the old-fashioned way, by hand. On my first day in the operating room, I used dish soap to scrub (there was no chlorhexidine or Betadine scrub solution with sterile brushes, as we have in the States). On my way into the OR, I scratched my left forearm on a nail that was hanging in the entryway; thankfully, my tetanus vaccination was up to date. After cleaning the wound and rescrubbing, I carefully entered the room, this time avoiding the jagged nail. I noticed a gecko crawling up the wall of the operating room. I was concerned about sterility as a contributing factor to patient safety, but with limited resources and no available alternatives, we had to make do with what we had. The following day, I observed the green operating room drapes hanging outside on a clothesline to dry, not exactly a routine step in the pathway to sterile processing.

The most amazing lesson that I brought back with me from Rwanda was the understanding of how one can communicate effectively in a time of duress without having to be abrasive. Most surgeons pride themselves on remaining calm during stressful situations, but being pleasant in their interactions is not always prioritized. At best, we may become short and to the point, usually leaving out a "please" or "thank you" because of our focus on the issue at hand. We tend to become frustrated if our needs are not met by our team, and some have been known to lash out at others. This type of behavior can often be counterproductive. While it may motivate people to move faster at times, it can also lead to anxiety and mistakes. The culture in Rwanda did not respond well to such tactics, something I discovered while caring for the young man who had been shot multiple times in the abdomen with an assault rifle.

We brought him into the OR, and the anesthesiologist intubated him as we prepped and draped his chest and abdomen in the usual sterile fashion. We performed an exploratory laparotomy through a standard midline incision, and upon entering the abdomen, we encountered a significant amount of blood. We needed to transfuse him with blood, which was available in the ER blood bank, but we did not have a large enough IV line to transfuse rapidly. In a tone that was abrupt and direct rather than friendly, I told the anesthesiologist that we had active bleeding and needed placement of a large-bore IV immediately in order to transfuse the patient more quickly. She did not respond, so I raised my voice. "Did you hear what I said? This man is bleeding to death and will die on the table if you don't get him transfused through a bigger line!" Instead of moving faster to place the line, she looked at me in shock. As I was about to begin yelling an insult, the intern said in a calm and pleasant tone, "Hey, sister, we have quite a bit of bleeding; would you mind placing a bigger line so we can get that blood in faster? Thank you." The anesthesiologist snapped out of the shock and immediately started placing the larger IV using the patient's neck vein. The patient had several injuries, which we repaired, and he survived, but no thanks to my method of communicating with the anesthesia team. This surgical intern, while lacking certain basic technical skills, helped save this patient through better communication. The culture in Rwanda was less tolerant of harsh words or abrasive tones compared to the United States.

While such toxic behavior in the OR may not provoke the same level of shock in the United States, there has been a gradual cultural shift, making improved OR etiquette increasingly necessary. The stereotypical surgeon who yells and throws instruments to get results is quickly becoming a thing of the past. A culture of civility has become the new normal, as surgeons who behave inappropriately are increasingly called out for their negative conduct by leadership as well as other members of the OR team.

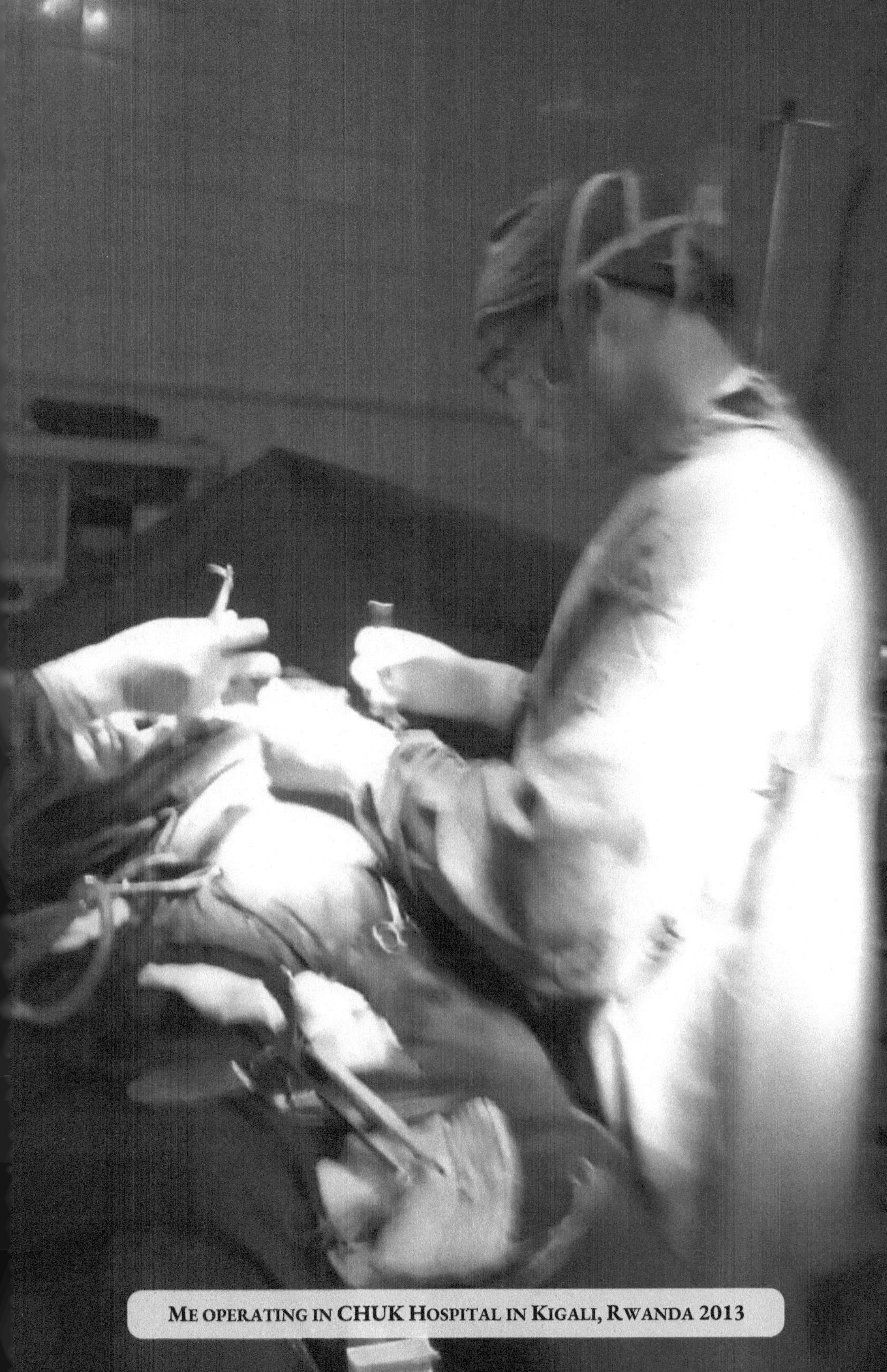

Me operating in CHUK Hospital in Kigali, Rwanda 2013

CHAPTER 18

Surgical Culture

Throughout surgical residency and many rotations at Johns Hopkins, the ICU was where I learned the most about taking care of some of the sickest patients outside of the OR. Even in the operating room, we are trained to listen to a patient's vital signs because our actions can immediately impact their physiology. The pulse oximeter constantly measures the patient's blood oxygen levels during the case and, while doing so, creates its characteristic beep with each heartbeat. If the oxygen levels begin to drop or the heart rate slows, the sound changes pitch and slows down. Such a change will immediately draw the attention of the anesthesiologist and the surgeon.

During laparoscopic surgery (in which a camera is inserted through a small hole), if the pressure within the abdomen from the carbon dioxide gas insufflated into it stretches the abdominal lining beyond a certain threshold, it triggers the vagus nerve to slow the heart rate. If I hear the pulse oximeter begin to slow while I am operating, I immediately look at the monitor to determine the heart rate. Many times, it is necessary to vent the gas from the abdomen to allow the heart rate to return to normal.

Most people consider surgeons to be the technicians of medicine, but we also have to learn a great deal about intensive care. By the time I completed my second year of surgical training, I had spent several months in the ICU and was well aware of what was expected for patients entering the ICU from the OR. When I knew that a patient would need to go to the ICU after surgery, I was expected to plan accordingly by ensuring that these patients had appropriate invasive lines placed while in the OR. This way, the patient could avoid being subjected to such uncomfortable procedures after surgery, having them placed instead while under anesthesia. It was considered poor form to bring a patient to the ICU without the lines placed, and depending on the ICU attending, you could receive a sharp reprimand if you did.

One day, I operated on a patient with pancreatic cancer whom we planned to admit to the ICU. The patient had a history of heart problems, and it was a long case. From the start, I knew that we were going to the ICU, and I also knew that my program director, Dr. Lipsett, was the attending that day. As we were about to begin the case, I spoke with the anesthesiologist about the patient, the extent of the case, and the postoperative ICU plan. He was aware of all these considerations but did not feel the patient needed an arterial line or a central line, both invasive lines used to monitor and support blood pressure. I voiced my concerns and told him I could place both lines myself before we began the case, but he insisted that neither was necessary. I pointed out that the ICU would not appreciate the patient arriving without at least an arterial line, but to no avail. "I've been doing this job far longer than you; we will be fine," he said, so I relented and proceeded with preparing the patient for surgery.

We completed the case without incident, and I helped transfer the patient to the ICU with the anesthesiologist. As we rolled into the unit, out of the corner of my eye, I saw Dr. Lipsett heading our way to see the patient. She watched as we entered the room, walked up to the patient's bed, and immediately recognized that there was no arterial line or central line. Without preamble to either of us, the first words out of her mouth, directed at me, were, "Why doesn't this patient have an arterial line?" The anesthesiologist was standing right there, but I suspect her tone may have intimidated him. He remained silent. I explained that I had planned to place both lines at the start of the case, but the anesthesiologist did not feel they were necessary. (Yes, I threw him under the bus in an attempt to save myself from her wrath. It did not work.) She said, "I don't care what he thought." She pointed her finger at him briefly and then turned back to me. Keeping her finger raised, she said, "If you knew what the patient needed, you should have placed the lines yourself. I don't care what he thought!" The anesthesiologist remained silent and suddenly found great interest in the patient's chart as we had our brief exchange. It sounds crazy, but I look back fondly on moments like this now because I know that they made me stronger. At the time, I was a bit embarrassed and felt foolish, but because of many similar episodes, and the irony of this situation, I can now see the humor in it.

The operating room remains something of a sanctuary in that it is one of the last places in medicine where there is relatively little regulation of what we do or say. This freedom can encourage those with a perceived God complex to misbehave when behind closed operating room doors. During my training at Johns Hopkins, I heard my share of yelling and even screaming in the operating room. Such behaviors were often directed at nurses, surgical technologists, or anesthesia staff. Some surgeons who seemed reserved and even pleasant outside of the operating room became completely different during an operation. It was as if a suppressed alter ego had been set free to wreak havoc. Aggressive behavior has thankfully become less tolerated over the years, but situations still arise where tempers flare. If things don't go as planned, there is always the potential for Dr. Jekyll to become Mr. Hyde.

For several years now, we have had a confidential online reporting system that allows employees to report patient safety or behavioral issues. All reported events are reviewed by the supervising staff and the chair of each department. This process allows appropriate measures to be taken, and feedback is provided to the reporter through the same online system. Such measures have resulted in a decrease in aggressive behaviors in and out of the operating room. Patient privacy remains protected, but the sanctuary behind the operating room doors is no longer a safe space for Mr. or Mrs. Hyde to emerge. As chair of surgery, I have had to sit down with several physicians to discuss reported events. Most situations involve surgeons losing their temper when they feel another member of the team is not doing something correctly. Instead of being patient and suppressing their frustration, they lash out. Now that surgeons are aware that unprofessional behavior can be reported, the incidence of such events continues to decrease.

When you have a system that works well, I am a firm believer in doing the same thing the same way every time. Dr. Cameron was very much a creature of habit, and he is one of the most successful surgeons living today. He often used the idiom, "Find something you love to do, and you'll never have to work a day in your life." He continued to operate until he was 80 years old and still participates in conferences and sees patients in the clinic because he loves what he does.

Dr. Cameron revolutionized pancreatic surgery, making Johns Hopkins a center of excellence for pancreatic cancer. The procedure for surgically removing pancreatic cancer from the head of the pancreas is called a pancreaticoduodenectomy, also known as the Whipple procedure, named after Dr. Whipple. Dr. Cameron has performed more Whipple procedures than any other surgeon in the world. He trained me and hundreds of other surgeons in the importance of perfecting what you do in the operating room through attention to detail, refusing to accept mediocre work, and demanding excellence. If you were more than one millimeter off from the intended area for your stitch, or if your needle was not completely perpendicular to the tissue plane, he would insist that you do it correctly. "Jeeeeeeeesus Christ! That's not perpendicular!" he'd say. "Take that stitch out and do it again!" While going through sessions with Dr. Cameron in the OR could be a bit stressful, it was an honor to be corrected by him. I know that sounds unusual, but it was like a rite of passage. You wanted to improve. You wanted every stitch to be perfect. Sometimes, while in the operating room, I and others who trained under Dr. Cameron joke that we can still hear his voice in our heads as we operate, demanding that every stitch be perfect. Most of his trainees have mastered the Cameron impersonation and have memorized many of his sayings: "Which side are you on, the patient's or the disease?" or "Why don't you just throw the patient down the elevator shaft?" These statements were used when the resident made serious mistakes, but thankfully I never heard either of them directed at me personally.

Besides the many hours spent with Dr. Cameron in the operating room, the lessons he taught outside of the OR have proven most inspirational. Although he was the most senior surgeon during my training at Hopkins, Dr. Cameron was consistently the first attending to arrive at the hospital every morning. For most attending physicians, the residents would have completed rounds on the service before the attending had even arrived, but Dr. Cameron often crossed paths with his team during rounds. Dr. Cameron had a tradition of taking the chief residents out for dinner at the exclusive Maryland Club in Baltimore several times each year. This is the same location where many of the American pioneers from Johns Hopkins' surgical past, such as William Stewart Halsted, Harvey Cushing, and Alfred Blalock, dined with their colleagues. We were honored to work and dine in the same spaces as these extraordinary surgeons who contributed so much to the field. At these dinners, Dr. Cameron shared many words of wisdom, but one that has most recently proven useful to me, which is in fact the very reason I have finally been able to write this memoir, is the lesson he taught us about how he succeeded at Hopkins.

When Dr. Cameron arrived at Hopkins, he was among a highly talented group of surgeons who, like himself, were skilled, intelligent, and deeply committed to the field of surgery. The very simple, but often underutilized, strategy he figured out early in his career and shared with us was waking up earlier than most to attend to important matters. The uninterrupted time early in the morning belonged to him, while most others were still sleeping. Although I achieved many of my goals without using this strategy, I still found this advice intriguing. I made a few half-hearted attempts to adopt this strategy around that time, but I found it far too difficult to employ during residency. It was too easy to hit snooze and get a few more hours of sleep rather than wake at 4 a.m. and begin working on a journal article or this manuscript.

Time is the most valuable asset we possess, and it is the one thing most people do not fully utilize. Many billionaires who built their fortunes themselves share this trait: utilizing those precious hours in the morning for their personal growth and productivity. Although I am very proud of the progress I've made in life thus far, I believe that if I had adopted this adjustment to my schedule earlier in my life, that time could have been used more productively.

CHAPTER 19

Pure Terror on Black Friday

The holiday shopping madness of Black Friday 2013 brought no interest to me. The only case I had that day was a laparoscopic colon resection with Dr. Marohn. The case was going fairly well, without difficulty, when my right eye started to fill with tears toward the end of the procedure. I didn't feel as though something had gotten in my eye, like an eyelash, and I certainly had not been splashed with blood. The tears started to run down my face as I thought, *What the heck is wrong with me?* I was slightly concerned that my tears would be seen by Dr. Marohn or other members of the team, but we were all actively working and looking at the monitor. After a few minutes, the tears started to dry up, and the case was almost done. Dr. Marohn scrubbed out of the case, leaving me to close the skin with the junior resident, whom I'll call "T."

After we finished the case, I told T that we should grab a quick bite before starting afternoon rounds, but a feeling of worry and distress consumed me. I was on call that night, and I knew that he was probably hungry, but I changed my mind and asked him if he would mind holding off on lunch until we finished the afternoon rounds. The uneasy feeling wouldn't go away. I just felt like I had to go home. After we dropped off the patient in the recovery room and gave a report to the nurse, we started to walk over to the surgical ward on the other side of the hospital to see our patients for the afternoon. Just before arriving there, my phone rang. Life as I had previously known it was about to change.

My 17-year-old son, Marcus, was always a good kid. He was often told he looked and acted a bit like Bruno Mars. He was the typical middle child, always looking for attention, a little on the histrionic side, and certainly the most like me in both looks and personality. He and I worked out together and would hang at home watching some of our favorite shows.

We were so much alike that we often came up with the same random thoughts at the same time, as if we were on a wavelength that nobody else was on. We're both a tad eccentric, and we really don't mind revealing our inner selves to others once we feel comfortable with them. Because he was so much like me, he also knew how to work my nerves.

We both shared a passion for music, but unlike me, he had a gift. He played several instruments and was self-taught. He carried his guitar everywhere with him. While Marcus had always been a good kid—really a saint if you compare him to what I was like at his age—his adventurous nature had often led to trouble for him on a small scale, up until that day.

I have come back to this part of my story several times and have had to stop each time. Even though it has been over a decade since the accident, it remains difficult to think about. I've had to internalize much of the pain I felt to keep it together and stay strong for my family. Reliving this moment takes a toll on me and has been the reason why this memoir has been placed on the back burner, year after year.

Not a single word can explain the sound I heard when I picked up the phone when my wife called that day. It was something worse than a cry, scream, or moan; it may have been some sort of combination of the three. In the most terrifying voice, Rosina cried out, "Something happened to Marcus! He's lying in the street, and he's not moving!" My heart felt as though it had stopped and then restarted at a rapid pace. "What? Was he hit by a car? Is he conscious?" I asked. With the same degree of terror and shrillness in her voice, she cried out, "Nooooooooooo, I don't know what to do!" I went into doctor mode. "Is the ambulance there? Is he breathing? You have to look at him and tell me that he's breathing!" She was frantic. "He's breathing, and we called the ambulance, but they're not here yet, and I don't know what to do!" I tried to remain calm. "You have to make sure that he is breathing, and if he isn't, you need to breathe for him. Check again and check his pulse." She said, "I can't feel his pulse." Despite the terror I felt as I ran through the hospital garage to my car, I knew there was a strong chance that he had a pulse, but because of the circumstances, she was not able to feel it. "Just make sure he is breathing. Is he breathing?" I begged. "Yes, he is definitely breathing; I can see his chest rise!" I then knew he had a pulse. Rosina put our oldest son, Tre, on the phone, and he reaffirmed that

Marcus was breathing and that the ambulance had just arrived. Tre, although terrified, was able to keep Marcus's head and neck stable while making sure that he was breathing until the paramedics arrived. By this time, I was in my car and on the freeway, driving as fast as possible.

Marcus had ridden his skateboard to his girlfriend's house and was on his way home with her when the accident happened around the corner from our home, just along the side of a nearby convenience store where there was a slight decline in the street. As they were coasting down the street, Marcus was distracted by a car that was driving toward them. He fell off his skateboard and hit his head, immediately losing consciousness. My wife and my other two children were home since it was Black Friday, and they had all considered going to the store to find deals. They found out what happened when Marcus's girlfriend ran hysterically to the front door, screaming for help. The entire family ran around the corner to see Marcus unconscious in the street. The paramedics picked him up and headed to the trauma center before I could get there, so I rerouted to the trauma center.

I arrived still wearing my scrubs and white coat. I frantically found my way into the trauma center's emergency room just as my son was being brought in by paramedics. Marcus was lying on the stretcher with his eyes closed and his arms in an extensor posturing position, which is an involuntary, abnormal position. They were rigidly straight and stiff, indicative of a severe head injury. He was not making any sounds and did not even open his eyes while the ER physician rubbed his chest and asked Marcus to respond. I watched from several feet away as a breathing tube was placed in Marcus's airway so that they could connect him to the ventilator to breathe for him. At the same time, they removed all of his clothes and started placing monitors and lines.

The trauma attending, a former fellow from Johns Hopkins, was someone I knew very well. He could see the worry in my eyes, and he knew that I understood how bad this was. They took Marcus for a CT scan of his head, and I was able to go into the room with him and watch from nearby during the scan. My fears were confirmed when I immediately recognized that there was a large amount of blood outside of the brain on the left side. The distribution of this blood was different from what I had expected, revealing a subdural hematoma rather than an epidural hematoma on the left side. Usually, epidural hematomas are arterial bleeds that rapidly expand and cause loss of consciousness after falls like the one sustained by my son, while subdural hematomas tend to expand more slowly because of venous bleeding surrounding the brain. Not all trauma patients present with classic findings, but with such a severe injury, the treatment was no different: emergent surgery.

Neurosurgery was consulted, and within an hour of his arrival, Marcus was taken to the operating room. There, the left side of his skull was removed so that the blood around his brain could be evacuated to control the bleeding and relieve the pressure. As the neurosurgery team operated on Marcus, my wife and I were in the family waiting area. We were in shock and had no idea what to do. Fear can be experienced in many ways by different people, depending on the circumstance. I have a personality type that always feels a need to look for solutions to fix problems, but I searched within and found nothing. I felt completely numb. Although my heart had to be going far above the normal rate, I was unaware of it. One of my biggest fears was helplessness, and it had me. I was consumed by the overwhelming feeling that I was trapped in a bubble where I had no control. I prayed for God's help as the neurosurgery team worked to save Marcus's life. For so long, I had depended largely on myself to get through difficult times, but this trial was far beyond my control.

I notified my program director, Dr. Lipsett, of what had happened so that arrangements could be made for the care of my patients at Hopkins. Behind the scenes, while we were going through the most traumatic hell of our lives, Dr. Lipsett went into action to give us more support than any other person, including our own family. My only expectation was for her to shuffle my schedule around to give me time away with my family, but over the following weeks, she went far above and beyond what was expected. Besides taking care of my schedule, she started organizing a schedule for residents and faculty to donate and bring us meals every day we were at the hospital. She also started a fundraiser and a blog for family and friends where they could donate money and receive updates.

Support continued to pour in from my colleagues. Dave Efron, who was the Division Chief of Acute Care and Trauma Surgery at Johns Hopkins Hospital at that time (he currently leads the Trauma division of the same hospital where Marcus was hospitalized), was the first member of our Hopkins family to arrive after Marcus's accident to show support. Dave comes from a family of surgeons and stayed at Hopkins as faculty after completing his residency there. He had, unfortunately, just been through a personal traumatic experience of his own, saving his wife's life after she had cardiac arrest in their home. As a trauma surgeon,

Dr. Efron has personally taken care of thousands of patients with every imaginable injury, but when your loved one is the patient, not everyone can keep it together enough to provide life-saving care like he did. I never saw Dave in a position where he portrayed himself as scared or uncertain; he was unshakable in my eyes.

Dr. Efron met us in the family waiting area while Marcus was in the operating room. He also contacted the chief of trauma, Dr. Scalia, who was with his family in Pennsylvania at the time. Dr. Scalia returned to the hospital and met us in the waiting area that same day to give his support. He assured us that Marcus was in good hands and that his team was there to provide him with all the help he would need. He did not need to do that, but this level of commitment to patient care is what makes places like Shock Trauma and Johns Hopkins one of the best in the world.

While waiting for Marcus to come out of surgery, Dr. Efron stayed with us. The hours passed like days until we got word that they were about to leave the OR. Dr. Efron and a member of the team escorted me to the CT scanner that was near the OR, where Marcus was to be taken immediately after surgery. They had removed the left side of his skull, but they had concerns that there could be blood on the right side as well. Sometimes, when both areas outside the brain have a bleed, the side with the larger bleed can hide a smaller bleed on the opposite side because of pressure. Such a bleed often declares itself once the opposing pressure is alleviated from the other side; missing a problem like that can be devastating if not quickly diagnosed. His neurosurgeon had seen these types of traumatic injuries enough times that he decided to take Marcus straight from surgery to the CT scan to investigate the other side of the brain. I watched as the images came up, and as I recognized the new problem, I became so weak in the knees that I almost collapsed if it were not for Dr. Efron, who had to physically support me. A large epidural hematoma appeared from an arterial bleed on the right side, which was pushing Marcus's brain over to the left. The team had to take Marcus back to the operating room to open the right side of his skull to stop the arterial bleed and remove the blood from that side.

I had kept my composure up until seeing the large bleed on the other side of Marcus's brain. I knew that this was not going to be good for his overall prognosis. All my hopes for a quick and easy recovery were obliterated. While outside the presence of my wife, I let my guard down and started to cry as I had never cried in my life. Having lost my grandmother, who raised me while I was in medical school, was horrible, and losing my father the year before was devastating. The thought of losing my own child was beyond what I could handle. Every ounce of my soul ached from the deepest part of my gut.

Dr. Efron held me and assured me that it was a good thing they found the bleed on the other side so quickly and were already headed back to the operating room to take care of it. He told me to focus on the good because I needed to stay strong for my family, so that is what I did. My wife was still in the waiting room, terrified. If I had lost my composure in front of her, it would have been more than she could have handled. I was able to stop by the restroom to run cold water over my face. I stared at my red eyes in the mirror and tried to will them to turn white again. I soaked a paper towel in cold water and gently pressed it over my eyes and forehead for a few seconds, then looked again. My eyes looked a bit less red, not great, but not as obvious that I had just broken down. I dried my face and regained my composure before returning to the waiting area to give my wife the update. I told her the news with a positive spin: the surgery team was worried about a possible bleed on the other side, so they immediately took Marcus to the operating room to take care of it. She was stunned and obviously concerned, but the slightly optimistic spin seemed to help. She didn't lose her composure as I had just a few minutes before. We waited again for Marcus to come out of surgery, praying that he was going to survive.

Marcus came out of surgery a few hours later and was taken to the intensive care unit. His surgeon came to the waiting room to update us on what they found and what was done during each operation. The left side had the bigger injury, a subdural hematoma, which they were able to take care of by removing the skull on that side, removing the clot, and controlling the bleeding. They expected more swelling after such a traumatic injury, so they left the skull off at the end and stored it in a freezer for replacement in the future. After such an event, there can be a bleed on the opposite side that declares itself only after the pressure has been relieved, so they routinely obtain a CT scan to look for such a problem. The large bleed on the right side was an epidural hematoma caused by a small arterial bleed, which was more straightforward to manage but did require removal of the skull on the right side as well. They controlled the bleed and evacuated all the old blood on that side. They replaced the skull on the right since the swelling there was not as severe.

Marcus' surgeon did not seem optimistic. He said that the next 48 hours would be the most critical for Marcus's survival and that he could not say much about his long-term prognosis. Marcus was breathing, but he still needed the ventilator. At that time, we did not see that our prayer for his survival had been answered; we wanted to hear that he would recover fully, but it was too soon to know the extent of his injury. As a family, we agreed that we would not cry in front of Marcus. We never did. Marcus had always been very sensitive to our family's emotions toward him, from a young age through his teenage years. If we laughed at him, rather than with him about something he did, he would get very upset. He did not want to be the focus of any joke at his expense. So, we agreed that if there was a chance that Marcus could hear what was going on in the room, we would not cry in front of him; we did not want him to be afraid. We agreed to share only words of affirmation regarding any good progress. I would cry alone, usually in the car; I did not want my family to see me lose control because I felt that I had to be strong for them. I buried so much of my emotion that even today there are times it surfaces when I allow myself to be vulnerable in front of others.

When we went to the ICU to see Marcus, he was still unconscious and on the ventilator, connected to numerous lines and wires. His head was wrapped in gauze, and an invasive monitor was inserted through the top of his skull into his brain to monitor the pressures. Hourly neurological checks were performed, which were necessary but difficult to watch because for the first 24 hours, there was very little neurological response to anything. When the nurses assessed his response to pain by pinching his chest, there was only a slight flexing of his arms. From a neurological standpoint, this was only a slight improvement beyond his pre-surgery state, when his arms had been extended. We were terrified that he would not come out of the coma.

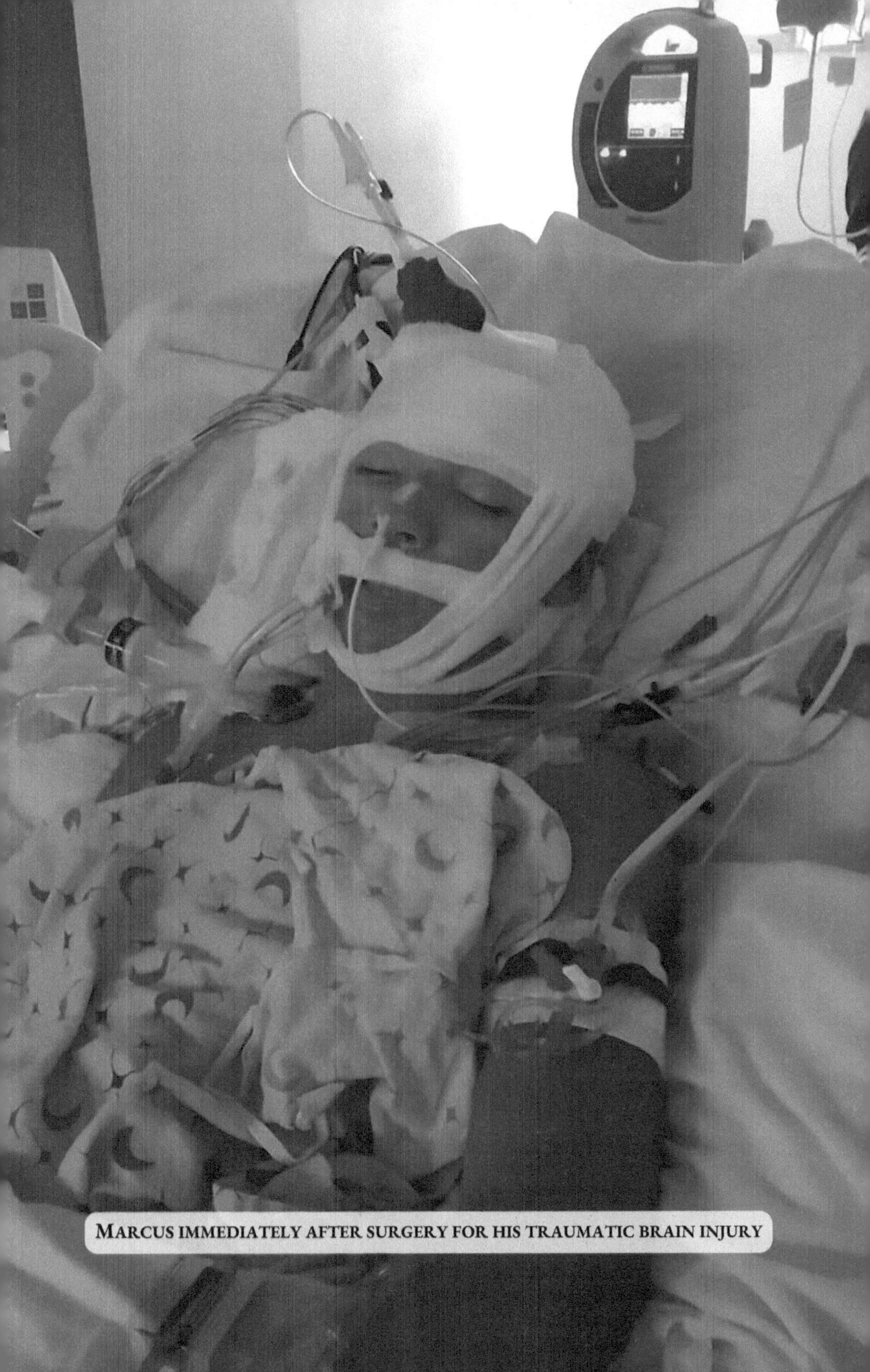

MARCUS IMMEDIATELY AFTER SURGERY FOR HIS TRAUMATIC BRAIN INJURY

I regretted not being involved enough in my father's care the previous year, even though I inquired about his status after he arrived at the hospital. After his death, I reviewed his medical records, obtaining all the details of his clinical presentation leading up to his passing. I often test medical students with the same clinical presentation my father had when he presented to the emergency room, prior to his death from an acute aortic dissection. Most of the time, they arrive at the appropriate diagnosis and request the proper workup—one that might have saved my father. The students are often shocked when I reveal that the clinical scenario was my father's. When they identify the correct diagnostic workup, which my father did not receive, I share with them that had they been on duty at the hospital where he presented, they might have saved his life. At the time, I had trusted the team to do the right thing and take good care of my father, so I didn't prod further about his clinical presentation or diagnostic workup. If I had obtained more information, perhaps I would have suggested the appropriate workup and prevented his death.

With this still on my mind, I was determined to do everything in my power to ensure my son would receive the appropriate care. Although the team that cared for Marcus was fantastic, I was resolute in not letting any negligence happen to him. Those feelings led me, at times, to become overly involved in his care. I was present at my son's bedside for most of his time in the ICU and participated in team rounds both as his father and as a physician. I respected the team and was very appreciative of their efforts, but I know I sometimes became too involved and overstepped.

On one occasion, Marcus was experiencing significant fluctuations in his blood pressure from periodic surges of adrenaline related to his traumatic brain injury, a condition called a "sympathetic storm." He was on medication to regulate his blood pressure, which would optimize blood flow to the brain. If the pressure was too high, he could rupture a blood vessel in his brain and bleed again, but if it was too low, his brain cells could die from a lack of adequate blood flow. Marcus had that invasive monitor that had been placed in his brain. His blood pressure required close monitoring so the doctors and nurses could appropriately adjust his medication to correct it. At times, he was on medication to lower his blood pressure, but at other times, they had to start a different medication to raise it. In situations where blood pressure is in flux, it is extremely important to obtain very accurate and frequent measurements using an arterial line. An arterial line is a bedside invasive procedure that entails placing a small catheter into an artery, usually the radial artery in the wrist. The catheter is connected to a pressure transducer, which shows continuous blood pressure readings on a monitor.

Marcus was having difficulty maintaining stable blood pressure. He did not have an arterial line, so the nurse had to use the blood pressure readings from an automated blood pressure cuff to manage his blood pressure. Because his pressures were so unstable, the measurements were not very reliable as minute-by-minute indicators of his blood pressure. If he had had an arterial line in place, it would have been a safer and more reliable way for the nurse to choose the correct medication and dose. The trauma ICU fellow was busy with other patients, so he was unavailable to place the arterial line when Marcus needed it. I had placed countless arterial lines over my years at Johns Hopkins, and although I didn't have privileges to perform procedures in that hospital, I was prepared to place the line myself if the fellow was not going to. I notified the nurse of my plan and asked her to pass the message on to the fellow. Just as I was about to place the arterial line myself, the fellow arrived and was able to do it.

In my mind, I felt that if something had happened to Marcus as I sat there and watched, it would have been my fault. Regardless of what hat I was supposed to wear, not acting would have been like watching a car drive down the street toward my son and not pulling him out of harm's way. At some point, my constant hovering became a bit overwhelming for some, and my friends and colleagues who visited could see the toll it was taking on me.

My research mentor and friend, Dr. Malcolm Brock, knew that my wife and I were sleeping in the ICU with Marcus for the first week. After visiting us one day and hearing that Marcus was starting to stabilize and was able to wean off the medication for his blood pressure, he paid for us to stay at a nearby hotel so we could get a good night's sleep and still be close by. At the same time, my program director, Dr. Lipsett, organized a list of volunteers from our Hopkins family to bring our family lunch and dinner every day we were at the hospital. Our oldest son had taken over the responsibility of taking our daughter back and forth to school, but we did not have to worry about food preparation because of the care and efforts of my fellow residents, faculty, and staff from Hopkins.

After a while, a member of the ICU team reached out to Dr. Lipsett and asked her to talk with me about trusting their team to do what was right for Marcus so that I could take a step back and wear the hat of a father rather than a physician. While I was a bit offended, they were wise to send someone for whom I had great respect. I explained some of my concerns to Dr. Lipsett and let her know that I would still speak up if something was wrong, but I agreed to tone down my constant hovering now that Marcus was no longer unstable. I know how Dr. Lipsett manages her patients in the ICU, and I have no doubt that she would have been at his bedside as much as possible if he were at Hopkins. At one point, I considered transferring Marcus there but didn't want to break the continuity of his care and possibly jeopardize his progress. Marcus had a great team who did an outstanding job, but any small problem can look like a major issue to the person looking through a microscope. Thankfully, Marcus became stable enough for me to step back and take the appropriate role as his dad instead of his physician. The road ahead was expected to be long, and my level of intensity was not sustainable. God had granted my biggest prayer of saving Marcus's life. Beyond that, we just had to keep up the fight and lean on God, along with the many angels who provided for Marcus and our family during the most trying time of our lives.

CHAPTER 20

The Aftermath and the Power of Music

Although my son could barely respond, he had stabilized and was transferred out of the ICU and into the step-down unit. He was not awake enough to protect his airway or eat, so after two weeks of minimal response, he had to have a tracheostomy placed along with a feeding tube. His vitals were all stable, his brain pressure monitor was removed, and he no longer required medication to regulate his blood pressure or the ventilator to breathe for him. He was still unable to do anything beyond opening his eyes and moving his left hand spontaneously.

Every night, I would sleep in the recliner facing Marcus's monitors. Rosina had a difficult time even looking at Marcus out of fear and anxiety that started immediately after seeing him unconscious in the street after the accident. Even after the paramedics had picked him up and were on the way to the hospital, she rode along in the ambulance in a state of shock, saying to the medic over and over again, "I'm going to die. I'm going to die." The medic told her, "You are not going to die." She continued, "Yes, I'm going to die. I'm going to die." The connection between a mother and child can run so deep that a child's severe pain or death can feel as though the mother has suffered the trauma herself. Rosina has always had a close connection between her physical and emotional well-being; emotional injury, for some, can manifest itself as real physical illness. She was so deeply injured by the thought of losing Marcus that she truly felt she was going to lose her own life. Even during the frequent neurological checks that were done by nurses to assess his response to pain, if I was not there, she would ask our daughter Danielle to watch and tell her what was going on. She slept in the back of the ICU, facing away from his bed, while I positioned myself in a recliner facing Marcus. After nearly one month in the hospital, Marcus was stable enough from a medical standpoint to be transferred to a facility called Kennedy Krieger for rehabilitation. In terms of what his mental capacity would be, it was too soon to say. From a functional standpoint, he was unable to follow any commands, he still had the tracheostomy, and he received all of his nutrition from a feeding tube in his stomach. The team told us not to be discouraged because his brain needed more time to recover.

Shortly after Marcus was transferred to rehab, the team briefly mentioned a traumatic brain injury (TBI) scale for determining his stage of recovery. It had eight levels, ranging from 1, which was no response, to 8, which indicated a purposeful and appropriate response. We were told that Marcus was at level 2 because of the non-purposeful movements of his left arm. They could not tell us whether his recovery would improve. "It is too soon to say," we'd hear quite often. We prayed for something. We were afraid that Marcus would remain in this vegetative state without any evident connection to the world. We did not know if he could hear us, and we did not want him to be afraid if he could, so we continued to avoid saying anything in front of him that could be discouraging. We talked to him and joked about things from the past as if he were engaging in the conversation. We prayed for something—just a sign that Marcus was still in there.

One night, Rosina had gone home while I stayed with Marcus. I was in my usual position, with my chair reclined, facing Marcus and his monitors, when I noticed his left arm moving a bit more than I had seen before. I jumped up and got close to him. "Hey, Marcus! Can you hear me?" I pleaded desperately, while at the same time begging God to give me a sign that Marcus was in there. Marcus raised his left arm above his head and dropped it slowly. "Marcus! Do it again! Lift your arm high!" I used my phone to record it this time, and he did it again. His response to my pleas was prompt and strong; there was no doubt that he could hear me. I asked several more times, telling him to wait until I asked him to do it again so as to prove it was not just a spontaneous movement. Marcus continued lifting his left arm, only on command. He started to tire after several rounds of this, so I told him, "You did great! It's okay to rest. You're going to be okay." That last part brought tears to my eyes. I was overwhelmed by the overall gravity of his condition, not really knowing if he was going to be okay, but also grateful that another prayer was answered. Marcus was now at level 3 of the TBI recovery scale: localized response. After surviving, the knowledge that Marcus could hear me and follow commands was another miracle that kept my spirit afloat until the next steps forward in his recovery. We were not prepared for the challenges that were to come.

It was, and still is, so difficult to think of who Marcus once was. Seeing pictures or watching videos of him before the accident is like looking at another person. Marcus was once the fastest kid on his track team and was excited about going to college the following fall. He was the most adventurous of all our kids and the most like me in personality. He wanted to be a doctor and would have completed medical school by now. It hurts to think of such things—so much potential, all taken away with a simple fall from a skateboard.

During Marcus's recovery, the downtime left me with much time to think, as there was little for me to do. We met other families throughout the process while Marcus was in rehab, and this brought some comfort in knowing we were not alone, though it was also challenging to see children in similar circumstances. My heart ached for those who were not following any commands. We felt guilty sharing the small improvements Marcus showed when talking with parents who were still desperate for any small sign that their child could hear them. At the same time, we felt envious of those who made progress much faster than Marcus. We understood that every brain injury was different, but we hadn't given up on the possibility that Marcus could have a full recovery. I felt myself slipping into a dark spiritual state but was afraid that if I showed my feelings to my family, I could drag them down with me. I was no longer grateful for the improvements we were seeing; I wanted a fully miraculous recovery. I wanted Marcus back. Instead of leaning on God and praying for ongoing improvement and strength for us to get through the difficult times as a family, I looked elsewhere for help. To stay focused and positive, I channeled my energy into researching clinical studies and emerging therapies related to traumatic brain injury.

Unfortunately, there is no widely accepted cure for traumatic brain injury (TBI) at this time—only supportive care. A plethora of animal studies exist, but nothing has come close to widespread clinical application for humans. Some invasive stem cell studies entail injecting stem cells directly into the injured area of the brain, but I was not willing to put Marcus at risk for a procedure that has little proven benefit and a high risk of serious complications. Despite my best efforts, years later we would fall victim to false hope surrounding experimental treatments of another sort.

While Marcus was about two weeks into his rehab, I had to prepare for my return to residency. There are extremely strict guidelines regarding specific requirements for surgical residency, with narrow windows allowed for time off beyond scheduled vacation. Fortunately, when Marcus had his accident, I had not yet taken my vacation. I used all my vacation time, in addition to the extra two weeks of allowed family leave, before returning. Although Marcus was still in rehab and was not making the kind of recovery we had hoped for, I knew it was time for me to get back to work, or I'd risk not being able to graduate on time. I met with our surgical program director, who agreed to allow me to return, but she insisted that I see a psychologist to clear me for duty. I took some offense to this at the time because I was so focused on ensuring my future wasn't impacted by my absence; however, she rightfully had to ensure I was ready to jump back into such a high-responsibility position. For an individual who has experienced the tragedy of a loved one's death or near-death, it can be difficult to fully understand the extent of the emotional impact.

As a chief resident, there was not only the expectation to perform technically challenging cases with an attending, but also the responsibility of overseeing a team of junior residents and their patients. At the same time, there was an expectation to take call and report for duty, often without sleeping the entire night. Amidst all of this, I also had to study for the annual standardized exams and mock oral exams. I thankfully had enough time off from these responsibilities when Marcus had his accident to begin learning how to cope with this enormous lifestyle change before returning as a chief resident. I did not need to utilize the therapist, although it would have been a reasonable option; instead, I talked with my wife every day and spent a great deal of time in prayer. Talking to a loved one may not always be the best solution for some, but it was for me. It was a way for us to support one another in our darkest hours. I felt like a part of my world was ending, and there was no other person I would have wanted to spend time with besides my wife. We had gone through the same horrible ordeal and needed each other to get through it.

Kennedy Krieger was a great choice for us, not only because of its outstanding reputation, but also because it neighbored Johns Hopkins Hospital. While Marcus was there, I was able to easily stop by during my breaks and after work to spend time with him. Marcus remained at Kennedy Krieger for several months on the inpatient unit. While there, he was cared for by a dedicated team of doctors, nurses, nursing assistants, and respiratory therapists. He also received physical therapy, occupational therapy, speech therapy, music therapy, and behavioral training support.

We were also recipients of care. They taught us how to take care of Marcus. During the first half of his stay, we held onto the hope that Marcus was going to make a full recovery while at Kennedy Krieger. As the months went by, we slowly had to accept that this was not the case. It was not until we had been there for a few months that we accepted we would have to learn how to bathe him. We had avoided this initially because Marcus was a teenager, and we wanted to respect his privacy. We believed that he would be able to take care of himself and that it was best for us to step out of the room whenever the staff was changing him. Once we accepted this reality, that we would be managing all of his basic needs, we began to fully understand the gravity of his condition and started learning how we would care for him at home.

We desperately looked for alternative therapies that seemed reasonable, since all the therapies thus far had not resulted in meaningful improvement. We had one positive experience with a nontraditional therapy for traumatic brain injury: high-dose fish oil. Some online stories advertised its use for traumatic brain injury, featuring one young man who was in a severe car accident with a very similar degree of injury to Marcus's. They started him on high-dose fish oil and reported dramatic improvement in his overall function. The story ended by showing that the young man recovered enough to return to high school for his graduation. Stories like this were so inspiring that we saw little harm in trying this regimen for Marcus.

Our former chair of surgery, Dr. John Cameron, had also seen this story at some point and approached me between morning rounds and conference to make sure I was aware of this treatment option. He even looked up the dose because he was so impressed with the apparent results. Marcus was not following any commands beyond the one episode when he lifted his left arm on command, but after being on the fish oil for only a few days, he started moving his left hand on command again. Next, he began playing thumb war and counting with his fingers. There were very few side effects besides the fishy smell and, later, some diarrhea, which eventually led us to stop it after seeing no further benefits after many months of use. But the initial miraculous changes that we saw opened our minds to alternative therapies.

In addition to being paralyzed on his right side and unable to provide basic self-care, Marcus still had a tracheostomy and a feeding tube, which my wife and I had to learn to manage comfortably. As a surgical resident in my final year of training, this was not a problem for me, but it was quite intimidating for my wife. She had to learn how to change and clean the tracheostomy and the feeding tube. The team was great about guiding her through the process, but this was a frightening aspect of his care for her. A mistake in managing a tracheostomy patient's airway could cause respiratory compromise if the tracheostomy fell out and was not replaced promptly. Losing the airway can lead to suffocation and death. This reality was overwhelming for Rosina. I was back in residency and in the hospital most of the time, so Rosina had to be the one to master these critical aspects of his care. My wife had to perform a tracheostomy change on him as part of the preparation for his discharge, and this was very difficult for her. She feared that she would be unable to insert it correctly and cause him to suffocate. Changing a tracheostomy often causes a patient to cough and even gag, so it can appear quite uncomfortable. Managing this aspect involved frequent suctioning when there was excess mucus in the airway and knowing how to change or replace the tracheostomy if it fell out or malfunctioned.

Before his discharge from rehab, he had to have another surgery at the University of Maryland to replace the left side of his skull, which had been left off and preserved at the time of his initial surgery to allow room for swelling. Now that the swelling had resolved, it was time to replace his skull, which meant he would no longer require the use of a helmet after it healed.

This was planned, and although we were scared, we were well prepared for what was expected. The surgery went well, and Marcus remained hospitalized for a few days afterward before returning to rehab. The rehab facility was somewhat reluctant to attempt removal of his tracheostomy due to the risk of an emergency, so we requested that the University of Maryland consider evaluating him for removal of the trach while he was under their care. Thankfully, Marcus passed his evaluation, which included capping the tracheostomy tube without any breathing problems, so we were able to successfully remove it while he was hospitalized for the skull replacement surgery. No longer having to worry about this aspect was a huge win. We had nursing care during the day to assist with his basic needs, along with therapists who would come once a week to continue his limited physical and occupational therapy. Marcus had started eating some food by mouth just before being discharged from rehab, but we were still dependent on his feeding tube for delivery of most of his nutritional requirements.

As Marcus's ability to use his left side improved and strengthened, a whole new set of challenges arose. Marcus maintained much of his baseline strength in his left arm, which was not far off from my own level of strength. Before his accident, Marcus was my workout partner. He and I would always go to the gym together and challenge one another. Despite being more than 50 pounds lighter than me, he could lift almost the same amount of weight. This strength made things quite challenging when Marcus was going through his aggressive stage of recovery, level 4. Even though Marcus could not use his right side and had very limited vision after the accident, he could fight off an army with his left arm.

He was evaluated by ophthalmologists, who did not think he had any light perception in either eye and stated that the brain injury involved the visual centers on both sides, so there was nothing they could do. We had spent enough time caring for him at that point that we could tell he had some vision in his left periphery, but because he was nonverbal, we did not know to what extent. We noticed that Marcus was more likely to behave aggressively if he was approached without verbal warning, especially when he was being changed or bathed. Bathing him was very difficult. Marcus would pinch, punch, scratch, and grab anyone within his reach. At times he put my wife into a headlock, and I had to pry his arm off her neck to stop him from choking her. The only way we were able to bathe him was to have one person responsible for holding his left arm while two others bathed him. While holding his arm, we also had to watch for his mouth. I lost track of how many times I was bitten. I have multiple scars on my right forearm from being bitten and scratched while trying to help bathe Marcus during the aggressive stage of his recovery.

As Marcus regained function and use of his non-paralyzed side, he would also grab at things attached to him, not understanding that he could hurt himself. While going through this phase, we had to use a restraint to restrict his movement, along with an abdominal binder around the feeding tube so that he would not pull it out. On several occasions, Marcus managed to get out of his restraint, maneuver under the abdominal binder, and pull out his feeding tube. When I was there, it was not too difficult to replace. On a few occasions when he pulled it out while I was at work, my wife was unable to get it back in. This meant taking him to the hospital to have it replaced, but by the time he was finally seen in the emergency room, the tract for the feeding tube had already closed enough to make it impossible to simply insert the replacement tube. He then had to undergo anesthesia to have the tube safely inserted, with a gastroenterologist performing an upper endoscopy to ensure proper placement.

Marcus didn't understand why he was fighting, nor that he was hurting himself and us while we were taking care of him. This is what we had to remind ourselves and others who helped care for him, so there were no hurt feelings when things got out of hand. This aspect of Marcus's care made it challenging to get him the help he needed. Most nurses were afraid to work with him unless I was present to hold his arm. Physical and occupational therapists were unwilling to make contact with Marcus out of fear of being bitten or grabbed. Before long, Marcus lost all physical and and occupational therapy sessions, and we went through new nurses and entire nursing agencies every other week. As we lost resources that we felt were necessary for his ability to progress in his recovery, we did the best we could to perform the various exercises and routines that we had seen his therapists use with him. We learned different strategies to keep ourselves and Marcus safe while maintaining some level of ongoing therapy.

On Father's Day of 2014, we all sat in the small living room that served as Marcus's bedroom. Marcus sat in his wheelchair beside Rosina, playing thumb war with his left hand. Thumb war became one of the first complex functions for Marcus to regain, and it also seemed to bring him joy. We often tried to get him to switch hands, but with the near-total paralysis still present on the right side, he was always reluctant to try using anything other than his functional side. Marcus was born right-handed, but after the accident, he not only lost most of the function on his right side, but initially didn't recognize his right side as being his own.

I am left-handed but, as I've stated, as a surgeon, I learned how to do most things with my right hand. When Marcus was around 12 years old, I started teaching him how to tie surgical knots with both hands while tying garbage bags. He thought it was fascinating that a person could train themselves to become proficient at performing difficult tasks with their non-dominant hand. Out of curiosity, he started forcing himself to eat with his left hand, just to see if he could do it. He began applying some of these same principles when playing the guitar. He played left-handed, like Jimi Hendrix, and also in the traditional style, in which he was already very skilled. Marcus was deeply committed to music and would stay up all night playing various songs until he had them memorized. He always had an excellent ear for music.

Even at the early age of three, Marcus showed that he had a finely tuned ear for music. The video game The Legend of Zelda: Ocarina of Time featured a musical instrument that players would play by pushing a series of buttons in a specific pattern to transport to different locations within the game. Each location had a corresponding cheat sheet, detailing the button pattern, allowing players to easily travel anywhere. As we played, I would look at the cheat sheet and then play the correct series of notes. One day, Marcus asked if he could try. We showed him how to read the cheat sheet, but instead, he played the correct notes for each location from memory. When this talent revealed itself further in his musical abilities as a child, we were not surprised. Marcus had an incredible passion for music, so much so that on that day, we began to understand its true depth.

On that Father's Day, about eight months had passed since the accident. We were all at home, and Marcus had only recently been released from inpatient rehab. He still had not been able to speak a single word up to that point, besides saying "no" and "yeah" with considerable prompting and without clear purpose. We were worried that he might never be able to speak again, but the recent addition of these two words was encouraging. It was similar to the first words of an infant. We were all sitting together in the living room, spending time with Marcus as he sat in his chair. After finishing several games of thumb war, my wife started humming and singing different popular children's songs, and to our surprise, Marcus started humming along. This continued for several minutes before we thought about playing some of his favorite music to see what would happen. Little did we know another miracle was about to take place. Marcus's favorite artist at the time of his accident was Jason Mraz. We put on one of the songs that we knew he liked, "I Won't Give Up." Marcus started to hum along with the melody, and as the main chorus began, Marcus hummed along and joined Jason, singing the tail end of the chorus: "on us." We all looked at each other and started to celebrate and shout, with tears in our eyes. That was the most we had heard from Marcus since the accident. Our excitement distracted him, so we all motioned to each other to be quiet and focus on singing the song with him.

I quickly began recording on my phone to capture the moment as he continued to sing most of the song. With his voice cracking in some areas, but also soft, Marcus sang, "I won't give up on us. Even when the skies get rough. I'm giving you all my love. I'm still looking up." Just like that, music became the key that opened the door to Marcus's voice. We have continued to use music as therapy for him. He still has difficulty expressing himself with open-ended questions, but he continues to make progress. He remembers songs from before his accident and has learned countless new songs since then. He is selective about what he likes and dislikes. He has a great time asking our Alexa device or Siri to play whatever song he is in the mood for. Whenever a song starts that he does not like, he tells Alexa to skip to the next song, and if he likes the song, he asks Alexa to turn it up. That may not sound like a lot, but for us, it is amazing.

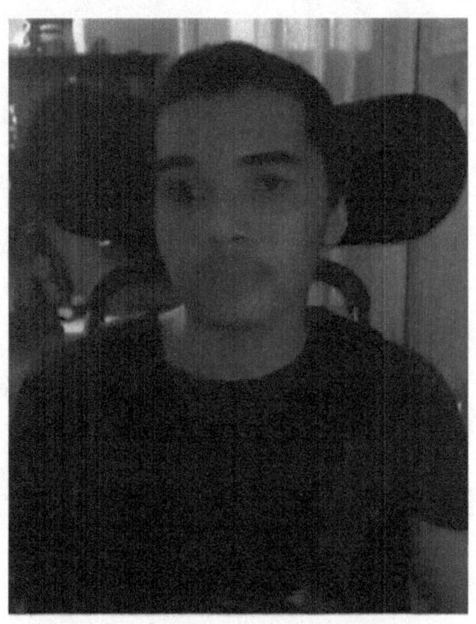

THE MOMENT MARCUS GOT HIS VOICE BACK AFTER HIS TRAUMATIC BRAIN INJURY, FATHERS DAY 2015

Marcus has had some difficulty regaining his ability to play musical instruments at the skill level he had prior to his accident, but this has not stopped him from doing the best he can, despite his vision loss and paralysis on the right side.

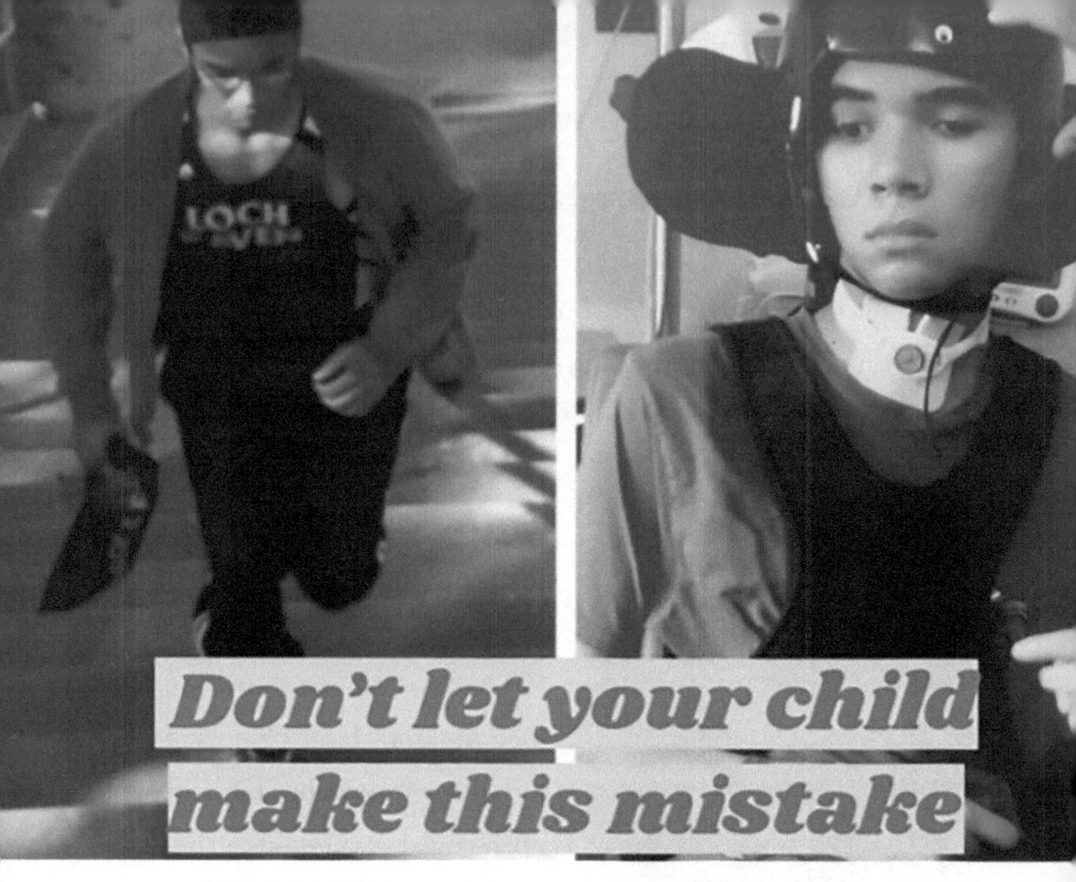

MARCUS BEFORE AND AFTER HIS TRAUMATIC BRAIN INJURY - A CAUTION ABOUT HELMET SAFETY

He can still play the piano with his left hand and remembers how to play the melody for several songs just by touch and sound. He received a harmonica for Christmas after the accident and figured out how to play it within minutes. He started off with "Jingle Bells" and worked his way up to Billy Joel's "Piano Man" after hearing it only a few times. He gets very excited when he learns a new song. He has even taught many of our regular nurses how to play some of his most common riffs on the piano, including "Boston" by Augustana and "Seven Nation Army" by The White Stripes. His passion and joy for music have helped him recover his ability to speak and regain part of the musical talent that we feared had been lost after his brain injury.

CHAPTER 21

A Kind of Monster

It is beyond unfortunate that some individuals in the world will take advantage of vulnerable people for their personal gain. After trying all available traditional therapies, we started looking for alternative treatment options for Marcus's traumatic brain injury. I found a research article that used a certain anti-inflammatory drug in patients who suffered from chronic neurological deficits caused by stroke, traumatic brain injury, and even Alzheimer's disease. What we believed at the time to be a potential miracle drug was marketed through online videos and real patient testimonials as a successful treatment for debilitating problems, but it was all an elaborate hoax.

Dozens of videos on the website for this treatment showed individual patients with significant speech, memory, and physical deficits. They received the treatment, and minutes after the drug was administered, they showed immediate improvement. One man who had a stroke was unable to say his wife's or children's names before the treatment. A minute after the treatment, he was pointing out each child and his wife, calling them by name. The wife and family showed their excitement and emotion—all captured on video. Another example was a woman who had a stroke. She walked in with a severe limp and used a cane. She also had significant speech deficits. Again, shortly after receiving the treatment, she started walking without a cane, her limp resolved, and her speech deficit improved. My scientific mind screamed to me that this was impossible. How could so many people be suffering unnecessarily if there was a miracle drug out there that could reverse their condition? I sought advice from several of my friends and colleagues who work in the fields of neurology and neurosurgery, none of whom had ever heard of this treatment. They, too, were very suspicious of these claims, but after watching the videos, they could understand my willingness to look into an alternative treatment.

I called the number provided on the website to inquire more about the treatment and the cost. The consultation and treatment were $8,000 for one visit. The company was using a drug that was sold in the United States for less than $500. The reason for the high price was that the drug had to be administered in a unique way, requiring administration by their doctor. In the videos, various patients were tested shortly after the drug was administered, and the apparent results, if genuine, were quite remarkable. It is beyond unfortunate that some individuals in the world will take advantage of vulnerable people for their personal gain. After trying all available traditional therapies, we started looking for alternative treatment options for Marcus's traumatic brain injury. I found a research article that used a certain anti-inflammatory drug in patients who suffered from chronic neurological deficits caused by stroke, traumatic brain injury, and even Alzheimer's disease. What we believed at the time to be a potential miracle drug was marketed through online videos and patient testimonials as a successful treatment for debilitating problems, but it was all an elaborate hoax.

As a surgeon, the idea of treatment with immediate results is not at all foreign to me. Many who choose a career in surgery do so because they can immediately see the results of their treatment after it is rendered. The idea of administering a medication in a special way to allow delivery to the troubled area seemed rational to me at the time. My logical argument against it was this: if the treatment really worked, why wasn't it already being performed all over the world by neurologists and neurosurgeons? A deeper dive revealed that the physician who invented this technique obtained a patent, preventing others from performing the treatment on patients without his permission. I thought that was the logical explanation for why someone would potentially withhold a lifesaving therapy from the world for money. Ethically, this goes against every ounce of what should motivate a person to be a physician, but unfortunately, greed drives pharmaceutical companies to drive up their prices all the time. I was going to access this therapy, while others who lacked the financial means could not. There were so many families whom we had met throughout Marcus's time at Kennedy Krieger who were in a similar state but could not take advantage of alternative therapies because of financial limitations. These treatments are not covered by insurance, so the cost was completely out of pocket. To

counteract this unfairness, I was committed to learning the technique—
if it worked—and then administering the medication to others who
needed it, free of charge.

I contacted the office for the initial phone consultation. I provided all
of our information regarding Marcus's history and all the traditional and
non-traditional options we had tried up to that point. I was a bit reluctant
to commit because of the lack of knowledge surrounding this treatment
among my colleagues.

I was warned not to trust this, but my mind kept going back to the
miraculous videos. I wanted to believe what I saw was real, and I was willing
to do anything I could to help my son recover. The day following my
phone consultation, I was contacted by the actual doctor from the video
who developed the treatment. He told me that most of his patients with
stroke and traumatic brain injury saw some improvement in their speech
and motor function after his treatment. He stated that the initial
improvement in the videos was only the beginning and that many
improved further without receiving other treatments. He even offered to
train me to administer the drug if I paid a training fee of $10,000. I could
then deliver this service to others but had to sign a contract agreeing to
provide him with a percentage of the profit. As shady as that sounds, I told
myself that this was a businessperson who had found something very
valuable and kept it to himself for financial gain. I thought that perhaps it
was all real and that the reason it had not spread like wildfire was because
the "doctor" was restricting its use to fill his pockets. The charlatan claimed
to cure diseases of the brain that have no known cure. My desperation led
me to believe this nonsense.

The media would have been talking about this miracle therapy for years if it really did what it claimed. I ignored the logic and put the ethical aspects aside by telling myself that if the treatment worked on Marcus, I would then learn how to administer it and provide it to others who needed it. The idea of him having a patent was ridiculous to me. As a surgeon, if I use a specific technique to perform an operation, I could claim to have developed it, but I cannot then stop others from using the same technique on their own. Yes, one could charge others to teach them how to do it, but after the knowledge is out there, a surgeon can do as they wish.

We paid the fee for consultation and treatment over the phone, bought the flight, reserved the hotel, and flew out to Florida with Marcus for this experimental treatment. I had watched every one of the dozens of videos I found about this treatment; each one was very impressive. No other treatment out there had even a fraction of the success. I believed so strongly that this was going to work that I ignored all the logical reasons why it was too good to be true. The doctor said that he was sure there would be some benefit for our son. I thought there was no way that all the patients and apparent family members from the videos could be paid actors. The claim that the treatment reversed permanent neurological deficits in patients with traumatic brain injury was what originally drew my attention to the research. Doing the same for stroke patients was a whole other level of extreme, but reversing the effects of Alzheimer's disease was such a preposterous claim that I should have closed the browser as soon as I read it.

We arrived at the office building, and the first thing they asked us for was payment up front. We gave them our credit card, and they "mistakenly" charged it twice, taking $16,000 instead of $8,000. They refunded the second charge after we recognized what they had done, but it took a few days for the funds to return to our bank account. I had only been a surgical attending for about a year at this point, so with all the other costs related to Marcus's care, we weren't exactly rolling in dough. Asking for payment before services were rendered gave us a bad feeling that something wasn't right, but we tried to stay optimistic. They ushered us to the back and had us watch a video highlighting many of their success stories, along with some international media coverage featuring a few patients from Australia who had used this treatment and recovered. After the video, they had us sign a consent form that read more like a waiver, freeing them from liability for any complications and not guaranteeing any results.

While waiting, the husband of another patient came to our room and shared his experience with the treatment his wife, who had suffered a stroke, was receiving. He stated that she had received several treatments and each time he noticed some improvement, so they were back again, all the way from Australia, for another injection. In the videos, there was no mention of repeat treatments. Something about the man seemed almost routine, as if he had gone through this song and dance many times, and he came off as a salesperson. At the same time, there was a sadness in his eyes that was a bit unsettling. I didn't know whether it was because his wife was still ill enough to require repeat treatment or if it was because he was being paid to lie about this fake story to influence others to proceed with the treatment. We thanked him for his time and expressed our hope that his wife would continue to improve as he stepped out. We expected to see him again at some point with his wife, but saw neither one, despite the clinic office being quite small.

We were then brought back to the treatment room, where Marcus was placed face down on the tilt-table gurney and positioned for the injection. With Marcus's inability to transfer from his wheelchair to the bed, this was not easy to do without our usual setup at home. Their nurse did not offer to help move Marcus, so my wife and I lifted him and, with some difficulty, managed to get him into the awkward position that was needed to administer the drug. The back of his neck was marked as the site of injection and then sterilely prepped and draped. My wife distracted Marcus to keep him still while I paid careful attention. If this worked, my plan was to say screw your patent and simply start helping people who could benefit from the treatment. The injection was administered, and he was then placed in the Trendelenburg position (on the tilt table with his head down). We anxiously waited for something miraculous, as seen in all the videos on their website. The doctor started asking Marcus questions, and when Marcus answered in his usual way, the doctor asked us whether that was something he had done before the treatment; it was.

After several minutes of questioning, there was no improvement that we could detect. We thought the doctor would have tested Marcus before the treatment, to be a bit more scientific about the approach, but this was not done. The only testing before treatment involved ensuring that we had the money to cover their fees and that our signature was on the consent form. The doctor stated that sometimes patients need to have a second treatment and that we could return another day to have this done, but they'd give us a discount for the next one. We were quite upset but remained hopeful that we might see some delayed effect or improvement from the treatment. It did not happen.

I had put so much faith in this treatment that I was blinded to what logic was telling me. If there were, in fact, a miracle treatment out there for such devastating problems as stroke, traumatic brain injury, and Alzheimer's disease, yes, it would be expensive, but it would be available everywhere. This doctor would not be wasting his time administering the drug himself in a small office. If the treatment reliably did what he claimed, he would have been a billionaire and would have had an entire network of centers focused on treating the masses. We left there feeling disappointed and swindled. We were prey to a kind of monster who targets the desperate. Not only did we spend a huge amount of money and time on a worthless treatment, but it was also incredibly difficult to travel with Marcus on a commercial flight. I felt especially devastated because I was the one who had found this treatment online and I'd truly believed that it was going to work. I was never the pessimistic type, but this bad experience pushed me into a dark place for some time. I keep a somewhat open mind but have remained afraid and reluctant to accept any nontraditional therapies since then. While the experience did not completely destroy my openness to new treatment options for Marcus, it led me to become much more skeptical of alternative treatments.

Sometimes it takes extreme suffering to level the playing field and show that we are all the same: vulnerable. Desperation does not always come to those with an abundance of material possessions. This is why, in the Bible, Mark 10:25 says that it is easier for a camel to go through the eye of a needle than for someone who is rich to enter the kingdom of God. Having money, power, and fame are all worldly, and such things can lead us to believe that we can do it all on our own, but this is just an illusion. At some point, we will all face struggles that can make all the material possessions we have amount to nothing. As dark as that may sound, it is sometimes the only way that all people, rich and poor, can find a path to God's grace. My suffering led to desperation for God. Once I hit my lowest point and was in the darkness, I looked to God to save me. My heart had become hardened from my repeated failures to fix Marcus's problems. I became so dependent on myself for a solution that I never looked to God for help. I believe that suffering is what truly led to my salvation. Suffering brought me empathy, thankfulness for all that I have, acceptance of my circumstances, and gratitude that my dark past does not define my future. Marcus, by the grace of God, has been a blessing in our lives and to others. His sheer joy, despite his severe disability, brings happiness to those around him. Every day, Marcus has to depend on others for all of his basic needs, yet he smiles. Marcus laughs, jokes, sings, and enjoys his time with others. How can I be sad? This world is temporary, and I believe that the time we have in this life is for learning lessons for what comes next. My son has taught me how to look at each day with thankfulness for what I have, rather than sadness for what I do not have. I still pray for ongoing healing for my son. I remain hopeful that he could someday have a miraculous recovery, but if this is not God's will, I will still remain faithful and appreciative of what God has given us.

CHAPTER 22

Back to Rehab

It was grueling, and wasn't getting much easier. After the failed experimental therapy, Marcus continued to go through an aggressive stage of his recovery. We continued having three people present to manage his bath time and other aspects of his care. The physical therapist had declined to work with him because of Marcus's violent tendencies to grab and bite. He had been making progress with regard to his strength, but when the therapy halted, he started losing out on potential physical gains. We desperately sought advice from his doctor at Kennedy Krieger, who admitted him again to the inpatient rehab to see if the right medication could help reduce his aggression. His aggression subsided a bit, but the medication made him too sedated to participate in therapies. We felt as though we were turning him into a zombie with all the medications. Despite multiple attempts to find a middle ground, we made little progress. After a few weeks, we were sent home with sedating medications to use when the aggression became too much to handle.

We tried our best to work with Marcus ourselves, but because of his lack of mobility, his left leg developed a contracture—a permanent bend at the knee caused by scar tissue around the shortened tendon—from diminished use. We tried multiple devices, such as braces, to keep the leg from developing this problem, but because of the behavioral issues, Marcus would not tolerate the placement of *anything* on him. Every time we struggled to get the brace on by force, he would rip it off. The only way we could keep it on was to restrain his left hand or sedate him, but neither option was appropriate on a regular basis. After several months of doing the best we could, our doctor from Kennedy Krieger recommended that we consider transferring him to a specialty center. She had gone to a conference where she heard about a facility in California that specialized in traumatic brain injury rehabilitation called the Centre for Neuro Skills (CNS). Patients participated in eight hours of various therapies, Monday through Friday, at their day program. After formal therapy sessions were over, the patients returned to the facility's apartment complex. There, they continued various therapies and received one-on-one care for those who needed that level of support. We thought the program sounded like a great opportunity but were concerned that they, too, would be intimidated by Marcus's aggressive behavior. We called CNS and shared some of the problems we were having, and they weren't unsettled by the challenges. They told us that this was common among their patients. CNS flew a team out from California to our home in Maryland to evaluate Marcus. Their physical therapist actually worked with Marcus despite being warned of his tendencies to grab, hit, and bite. She positioned herself so that she was able to safely transfer him from his bed to his chair, all by herself, without being attacked. We hadn't seen this in months because of Marcus's aggressive behavior. At one point, Marcus did grab the back of her shirt, but she was able to talk him down and relax him enough for her to break free without incident. She emphasized, "This is routine for us." The program accepted Marcus, and our insurance approved his admission. A few days later, we packed his belongings and flew out to California to spend the next several months enrolled at CNS.

The trip to California with Marcus was a challenge in itself. The transfer from the wheelchair to the small airline seat was difficult. Some individuals cannot or should not come out of their wheelchair because of the significant support their bodies require. For those who need constant attachment to a ventilator, such a transfer would be impossible without medical transport. While Marcus was able to support himself fairly well in a normal seat, keeping him there required constant monitoring and attention. We took turns being on constant duty, making sure he didn't unbuckle his seat belt or reach into the aisle to grab people passing by. Marcus has a habit of slapping butts that are within reach, and he doesn't discriminate whose butt it is—male or female, mom or dad, cat or dog. If you have a butt within Marcus's reach, it is getting slapped. Most people are understanding when we are unable to stop him in time, but every once in a while, someone reacts harshly despite the obvious fact that Marcus has a disability.

In some ways, it's a blessing that Marcus is unable to walk around freely at this point in his recovery. Sadly, many people who have suffered from a traumatic brain injury have disabilities that are not easily visible. Some look like anyone else and are able to walk around on their own without assistance, but they may at times have a lapse in judgment that leads to significant conflict. At worst, there have been incidents that resulted in horrible tragedies such as assault, arrest, or even police-related shootings. Since Marcus has not yet regained enough mobility to walk and still has significant visual loss, we don't have those fears for him at this time. However, it wouldn't be hard to imagine a future scenario in which he could get in trouble for grabbing or touching someone inappropriately. We managed to get through the entire flight without an incident; all butts were safe and accounted for.

When the plane landed, getting Marcus back into his wheelchair was tough. The aisles were very narrow, so I had to transfer him to the airline's smaller wheelchair first, as I'd done when getting him onto the plane. We intended to do the same thing with the help of a few airline staff members assisting, but Marcus was so frustrated and uncomfortable by the end of the flight that he was agitated. I was worried that he might bite or grab one of the assistants during the transfer, so I decided to pick him up myself, walk him down the aisle in my arms, and then place him directly into his chair. I have tried to stay in shape and work out regularly, so picking up Marcus's 155 pounds was not the issue. Immediately after picking him up, he screamed and then clamped down, biting my shoulder and simultaneously pinching my chest as I carried him down the narrow corridor. I endured the pain and managed not to scream or drop him while I wobbled with him in my arms as he continued to clamp down. I reached the wheelchair in what felt like minutes but was likely only a few seconds and placed him into the chair before he drew blood. I was bruised, with a full impression of his teeth etched on my shoulder, but not badly injured.

We got Marcus safely to CNS from the airport, where we were met by a small army of staff members who introduced themselves and immediately took control. We were unsure whether they would be able to handle Marcus, especially after the experience we had on the plane. He was upset and ready to fight. The team struggled at first, but their care and compassion, despite Marcus's aggression toward them, were obvious. It took several team members to accomplish their goal of bathing him that day, but they got through it without any injuries. We stayed with Marcus as he adjusted to the new place and routine. I was thankfully able to take my vacation, which gave me a few weeks to help with the transition. The amount of therapy was intense, but the immediate immersion led to a much faster adjustment to the change. Marcus ripped several shirts off some of his therapists, and one therapist even had her finger bitten by him, resulting in a fracture. Despite such extreme circumstances, they all remained professional and never took out their frustration on him. When such things happened, they blamed themselves for allowing the injury to occur because they knew what Marcus was capable of. It is hard to find such special people in healthcare who are willing to put themselves in harm's way in order to help their patients.

After a few months of intense therapy, the aggressive behaviors were finally extinguished. The therapists were able to develop a system that gave Marcus the freedom to show that he was upset without hurting others. When he would get frustrated about something, instead of trying to force the issue immediately, they would simply say, "Let us know when you are ready," and somehow this de-escalated his anger by letting him know he had control. Usually, this led to a very brief pause in his care, such as brushing his teeth or bathing, but he would then allow his care to resume after a minute. Tackling the aggressive behavior allowed us to start learning how to care for him without worrying about our own safety or the safety of others. Toward the end of his time at CNS, each of us in our family, including our youngest daughter, was able to assist him in transfers and with certain daily care activities.

After Marcus made some progress, we were able to bring him back home. We had flown back and forth several times from Maryland to California while he was in rehab. The day we arrived to bring him home, we decided to walk in quietly to see whether Marcus could recognize us. We had been told by ophthalmologists that he was blind, and that the limited light perception he had from his left lateral side was not enough for functional vision; we did not believe this. We hoped and prayed that his vision would improve and that he perceived more than just light. As we walked into his living quarters, we motioned to his nurse that we didn't want him to hear us. My wife tiptoed up to his left side, where we knew he had some light perception, and got close to his face without saying anything. There was a brief pause as he looked straight at her and exclaimed, "My mom! My mom!" Rosina embraced him, and he wrapped his functional arm around her with so much joy. There is no doubt that God is good, and if He healed the blind at the time that His Son walked on this earth, we hold onto the belief that miracles still happen and pray that, God willing, Marcus's vision will continue to improve.

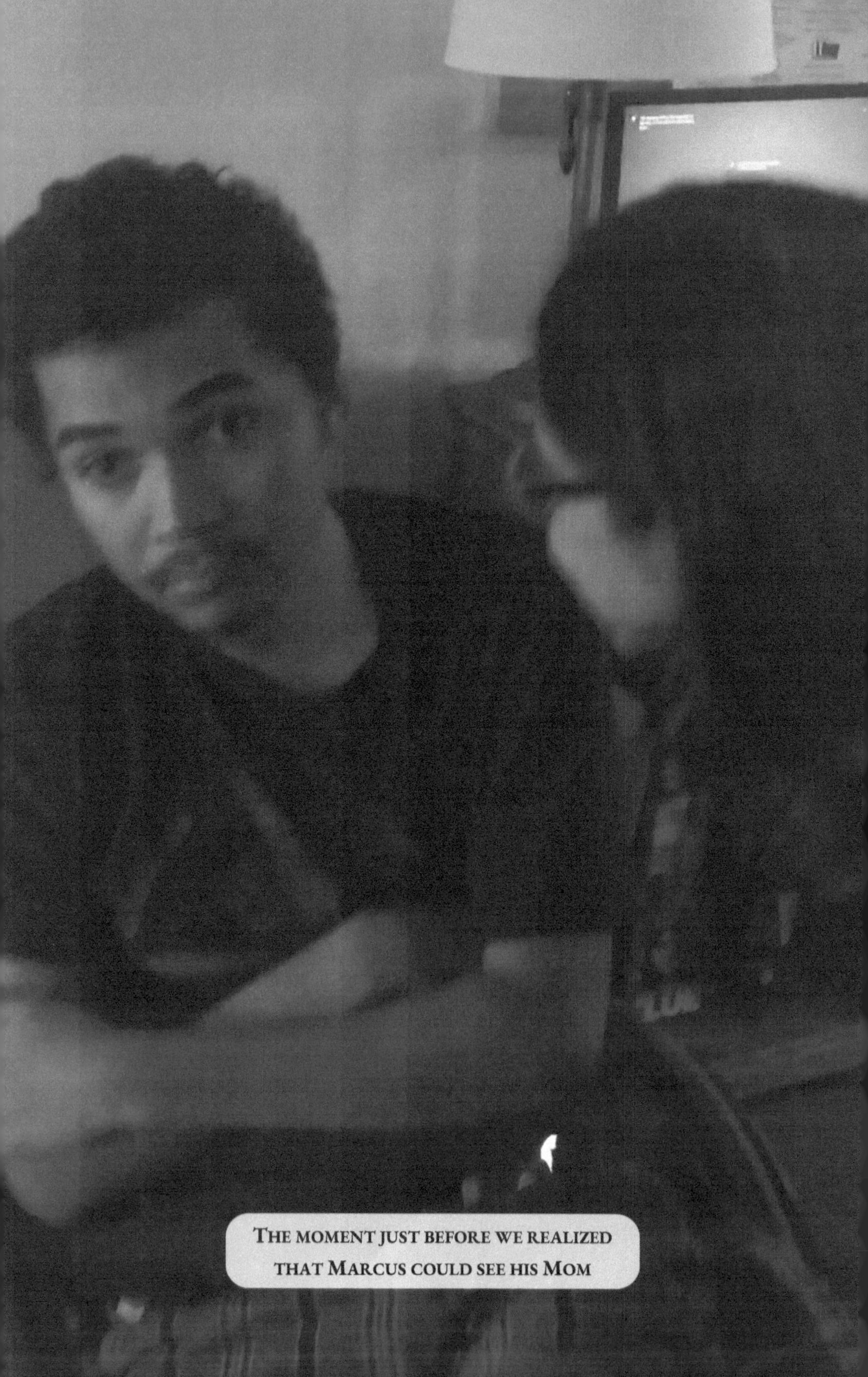
THE MOMENT JUST BEFORE WE REALIZED
THAT MARCUS COULD SEE HIS MOM

We flew back home with Marcus and started working on arrangements to find home health nurses who could help us. People who work in patient care can be some of the most caring and wonderful individuals in the world, but in all professions, there are also many who go into the field for the wrong reasons. Some couldn't care less about the importance of what they do and the people they are caring for. It doesn't matter whether you are a physician, nurse, nurse practitioner, nurse assistant, physical therapist, or in any other patient-care-related role; your responsibility should be focused on the patient. We have been fortunate to have found a number of excellent nurse assistants to help us in our home with Marcus over the years, but we have also encountered many who have made life very challenging for our family. Unfortunately, some home care nurses look for opportunities to have a job where they can simply sit down and watch television or play on their phone while they are supposed to be caring for a human being who needs it. Some have even fallen asleep while with Marcus. Patients who have no family member to advocate for them can end up with a home care nurse who is not providing appropriate care, and they are neglected.

We have been fortunate in that my wife hasn't had to work since Marcus's accident, so she has been available to ensure that he has been well cared for. Due to Marcus's traumatic brain injury, his cognitive functioning is now at the level of a four-to-five-year-old, but he has a grown man's body. With his inability to walk because of right-sided paralysis and his vision loss, he needs considerable help with all his basic needs. Moving him from the wheelchair to the bed or to the toilet is not an easy task for one person, especially if Marcus outweighs you. Rosina has always been there for Marcus, but when I am at work and his nurse doesn't show up, Marcus still needs to be cared for. She has sacrificed her body and has been injured on multiple occasions when she was left with no other option but to care for him by herself. Patients who do not have a loved one caring for them can be left in bed until the next shift arrives, often hungry, thirsty, soiled, and alone. These are the patients who often develop pneumonia, bedsores, blood clots, malnutrition, dehydration, and other preventable health problems while in their own home. Thankfully, because of Rosina, Marcus has never suffered from any of these problems.

We have had home care nurses who routinely come late or do not show up, often without excuse or even notification. Some come in for their shift but are determined to do the least amount of work possible before leaving. One of our earlier home nurses often worked the night shift elsewhere, so while she was with us, we would find her asleep while "taking care of him." Another had been going outside to smoke while we were out shopping; we only found out about this when she called us back home because she accidentally locked herself out of the house. When we arrived, we found that she had first tried to break in through the front door and had damaged the handle with a screwdriver before finally calling us. Another nurse would take up space on the main couch in front of the television and lay out her belongings on each side of her so that she had the entire couch to herself. The worst have been those who are rude and cold to Marcus; we part ways with them as soon as they are identified. Negative people have a negative influence on those around them, and Marcus is vulnerable in many ways because of his brain injury. If he is treated poorly, he can react negatively with aggressive behavior and may even become physically aggressive toward the person he is upset with. He unfortunately still has expressive aphasia, meaning he cannot always say what he may be thinking. He understands quite a bit, but he still does not possess the ability to communicate his feelings or needs. He also has memory problems, so he may not remember certain things that have happened recently. This scares us when there are concerns about mistreatment because he cannot tell us what happened. When in doubt, we don't leave Marcus alone while under their care until we can find a replacement whom we can trust.

Some of the hardest moments have been when Marcus was neglected and physically harmed. We pay close attention to every aspect of his care and look for both physical and behavioral signs of abuse. People who cannot speak for themselves because of physical or mental disability are unfortunately often the targets of evil, malicious individuals who place themselves in caretaker positions so that they can fulfill whatever sick fantasies they may have. We had to take Marcus out of one of his first day programs after we found that he had a bruise on his left chest that left the imprint of two fingers around his nipple, as if he had been pinched. We were called and notified that Marcus had been upset for no apparent reason and had ripped his own shirt. We picked him up and found these marks on his chest. We questioned the staff about this and were told he had done that to himself with his right hand, which happens to be his paralyzed side. His right hand was barely able to grasp a potato chip, let alone pinch himself hard enough to leave a bruise. An investigation didn't turn up enough evidence to find any of the caretakers responsible. We moved on to another program that had its own set of issues.

The new place seemed appropriate at first, with a welcoming staff, but they had a policy that did not allow family members to stay to help orient the caretakers to the patients' specific needs. We thought perhaps this was for the confidentiality of other patients, so we did not question it. One day, my wife received a call from this facility telling her that Marcus had managed to grab a pen from somewhere and used it to release his seat belt. He somehow fell to the carpeted floor and sustained an abrasion to his forehead. We were upset, but we thought that their description of events leading to this was not too far-fetched. Marcus always looks for opportunities to take his seat belt off, and we know that he can do so if given the chance; we never allow him access to anything that can serve as a key, such as a pen, without supervision. We'd warned his caretakers that they had to be sure to keep objects like that out of his reach, but mistakes can happen.

We decided to give the facility a chance and spoke to them about the importance of close supervision and preventing falls. Falls can be very dangerous for people who have had traumatic brain injuries, so this was a situation we insisted could never happen again. He had never fallen on our watch, and unlike at home, they had a full staff with backup care providers for lunch and bathroom breaks, so Marcus should never have been unsupervised. Things had been going well until a few months later, when we received another call from the facility stating that Marcus had once again taken a pen from an employee who was covering a lunch break with him and released his seat belt. He then allegedly threw himself out of his chair, but this time they claimed that his care provider leaped forward to catch him as he fell. They apparently bumped heads, and

Marcus fell on top of him. They said he was fine and only had a small bruise on his face. When Marcus arrived home, we not only found that he had a bruise on his face, but one of his front teeth had fractured in half. We called the facility, and they claimed they believed he was already missing that part of his tooth, so they did not mention it to us when they called. We lost all trust and again took him out of the day program.

It hurts to see harm done to a child, let alone one who is defenseless and unable to communicate what happened. We kept Marcus at home during the day for several months until we found another adult day care program that we could trust. Many programs seem to focus primarily on money rather than patient care. Each patient they add to their center puts more money into the owner's pocket. Hiring more staff or paying competitive salaries with benefits to ensure high-quality care does not seem to be a priority for some adult day care centers. If someone is unable to communicate well, their families may never know what conditions are like for their loved ones while they are there. Some centers had only one main room crowded with patients with disabilities and special needs, and just a few caretakers supervising the entire group. Most of these patients were in wheelchairs, but some were also ambulatory and could very easily leave unnoticed. Places like this can thrive because most, if not all, of their clients are unable to communicate effectively with their families due to their disability.

Learning to Tap

Sometimes, the doctor needs to be the patient. I've been seeing patients in my clinic who have been getting younger and younger each year with colon cancer. Not long apart, I saw a young woman in her late twenties with an obstructing colon cancer and then a young man in his late thirties with the same condition. I have a family history of colon cancer, so this inspired me to get my first colonoscopy when I turned forty. I happened to run into one of the gastroenterologists to whom I regularly refer patients while I was rounding in the hospital. I asked whether he could work me in for a colonoscopy, and he found a slot for me within a couple of weeks. The process was what I expected it to be. The outcome with respect to what he found, however, was not. "It took me quite a while because you had over twenty-five polyps that I had to remove." I was still a bit out of it due to the anesthesia when he told me this. Despite my confused state, this got my attention. He provided me with color pictures and his dictation of his findings. The pathology was going to take a few days to come back, but he suspected that many of these were adenomas. Adenomas are benign, but they are the type of polyps that can turn into cancer over time. Thankfully, he was very thorough and felt he removed all of them, but despite this, he advised that I repeat the colonoscopy in a year, just to be safe. I chalked this whole thing up to being a fluke, but obliged and repeated the colonoscopy with him the next year.

The next year came along quickly. My life remained pretty much unchanged during that time. My diet wasn't great. Red meat and processed foods were the foundation of my diet. I was obese, out of shape, and didn't care very much about what I was putting in my mouth. No foods were off-limits.

I had not made my follow-up appointment yet, but again saw my gastroenterologist while I was rounding in the hospital. It was so strange to say "my gastroenterologist." He got me back on the schedule, and I had my second colonoscopy a few weeks later. I was not very worried and expected all to be well, considering I had just had all the polyps removed only a year earlier. However, all was not well. My gastroenterologist found another five polyps, one of them over one centimeter in diameter. The pathology all came back the same: adenomas. Any one of them could have gone on to form colon cancer. This was not normal.

Thankfully, he again removed all of the polyps, but this time he urged me to see a geneticist to rule out an underlying mutation that I could have. He also scheduled me for another colonoscopy in a year.

This was before the late actor Chadwick Boseman died. He had been in the prime of his life and completed *Black Panther, Avengers: Endgame,* and other films while being treated for metastatic colon cancer. Unfortunately, I had many patients who were his age and younger who were fighting the same disease. With my family history of colon cancer and these rapidly recurring polyps, I was prepared to make some changes in my life.

I saw the geneticist, who performed a complete array of tests to look for any mutations that could contribute to all the polyps I had formed. I was convinced they would find that I possessed some rare mutation, like Lynch syndrome, that would destine me to develop colon cancer. I had even started prepping myself for the possibility of a prophylactic, or preventive, total colectomy.

This is a concept similar to a prophylactic bilateral mastectomy for someone diagnosed with a BRCA mutation as a way of significantly reducing their risk of developing breast cancer. If I had such a mutation, I would also have to warn my kids so that they could be evaluated to determine whether they also carried the gene. It took several weeks for the genetic results to be finalized, and they were all negative. Although this was a huge relief, I now had to shift my concerns to the question of why. If not a mutation, what could explain why this happened?

Sometimes, there is no answer to the question of *why*. While I do have the ability to let go of things that don't matter, I was quite committed to figuring this out. The one variable that I had not attempted to alter was my environment. Both what I exposed my body to and my my general state of health were not optimal. I had just shy of a year to attempt to improve my health through diet and exercise before the next colonoscopy would reveal whether I could make a difference. Certain factors can reasonably be assumed to cause cancer that cannot be explained by genetics.

When you look at certain populations, you may see a low risk for certain types of cancer, but when those individuals are placed in another environment, the incidence of cancer often increases to mirror the new environment in which they live.

The power of science cannot be ignored. Many adverse health conditions don't just appear. Most people readily accept that smoking causes lung cancer, understanding that exposing the lungs to the chemicals found in cigarettes can lead to cancer. Why is it so hard to believe that exposing the colon to chemicals found in some foods can do the same? I would argue that the obesity epidemic in the United States is an even bigger problem than smoking.

There is very little regulation regarding what we regularly expose ourselves to each day. Unlike cigarettes, which carry a warning on every pack about the known risks, such warnings do not exist for food. Some foods have a shelf life of well over a year. This is not natural. For a food to have such a long shelf life, there is often some process that makes this possible using various chemicals to extend its life. It's good for business, but not for consumers. These chemicals must be processed by our bodies, and this exposure is analogous to smoking cigarettes. The cells lining our colon, when exposed to such chemicals over time, can experience damage to their DNA. Damaged DNA can lead to mutations. Mutations can lead to cancer.

With this knowledge, I chose to perform an experiment on myself: for a year, I removed more than 90% of processed foods and red meat from my diet. This process took some trial and error, but the prospect of making a significant difference in my health was a strong enough motivator for me to follow through. I also started to exercise regularly. As a busy surgeon, time was not readily available, so I had to make more time. I began waking up earlier to fit this new routine into my schedule without taking time away from my family when I got home from work. With these additional changes, I started to lose fat and gain muscle. In one year, I was in the best shape of my life.

I had my third colonoscopy, and there were no polyps. If my diet and exercise could have such a positive impact in this regard, there are most certainly many other beneficial, perhaps unseen, effects occurring systemically. Although I have never had heart problems, issues that contribute to heart disease slowly accumulate over time. Small positive changes over time can be protective and preventive for overall health. Obesity increases your risk of heart disease, cancer, and stroke. These were the top three causes of death in the United States before the COVID-19 pandemic. With the advent of COVID-19, it rose to become one of the top three causes of death in the United States, displacing stroke in 2020.

While death is inevitable, it often occurs at an earlier age for those who are obese. We had a close family friend, a physician, who had worked hard all his life to get to where he was. He had his own practice, a wife, and kids. He was obese and in his early fifties when he decided to get into shape. Unfortunately, much of the damage had already been done before he began making changes to his health. He had underlying coronary artery disease from many years of unhealthy eating and high cholesterol and suffered a heart attack while working out at the gym. He spent years telling his patients what they needed to do to help themselves but waited too long to follow his own advice. I am not so different from our friend; my health, in fact, was being affected by my diet. I was obese and eating many of the foods that I advised my own patients against eating. If I had not been fortunate enough to get the colonoscopy when I did, I could very likely have had colon cancer by this time and suffered the same fate as the late, great Chadwick Boseman. Chadwick was unfortunately diagnosed with colon cancer after it had already spread, and despite his youth and aggressive treatment, it was not enough. There is only so much that we can do to prevent some things from happening, but for what I *do* have control over, I intend to do my best to optimize my health.

My other motivation for getting in shape was to improve my strength to help Marcus. I lift our son every day from his bed to the wheelchair and back. In the past, I'd hurt my back and shoulders at times during these lifts. While these injuries were mild, I wanted to increase my strength to mitigate the risk of such problems as I age. I was always afraid of certain exercises, such as the deadlift and squats, but after doing some research, I found that these two exercises, if done correctly, could significantly improve my overall strength and ability to safely lift my son. I started off with low weight, focusing on form, and sought the help of personal trainers to ensure my technique was correct. Over time, I slowly increased the weight or repetitions with progressive overload, and with that, I saw increased muscle mass that I had never achieved in the past.

In the past, I was never interested in working my lower body because, aesthetically, it was always hidden by clothing, so I didn't appreciate the reasoning from an overall strength standpoint. Studies have shown that the squat and deadlift cause the biggest boost of natural testosterone production. By implementing these key exercises into my routine, I started seeing progress not only in my lower body but in my upper body as well. Having a more balanced regimen allowed for a stronger foundation for bigger lifts and more efficient muscle gains. Many of the aches and pains that I felt in my lower back became much less common.

The most difficult challenge was finding the time for exercise with my busy schedule as a surgeon, a husband, and a dad. I started by working out after we got Marcus to bed but felt guilty taking time away from my wife. This time was usually spent catching up on the day's events and watching TV. I eventually accepted that the best time would be in the morning, before work, while everyone was asleep. The challenge was making it a habit. I found early on that excuses are often easy to come up with as a way to justify or rationalize why I should skip a day and sleep in. I found it much harder to allow such excuses if I planned the workout session in advance. If I planned which exercises I would do the next day before going to bed and prepared my pre-workout meal, there was a much better chance of sticking to it. Planning for success with big goals is important, but it also works for smaller goals. What may seem like small wins can, over time, add up to be quite significant. This method of working out every morning not only became a habit but also something I very much enjoyed and looked forward to.

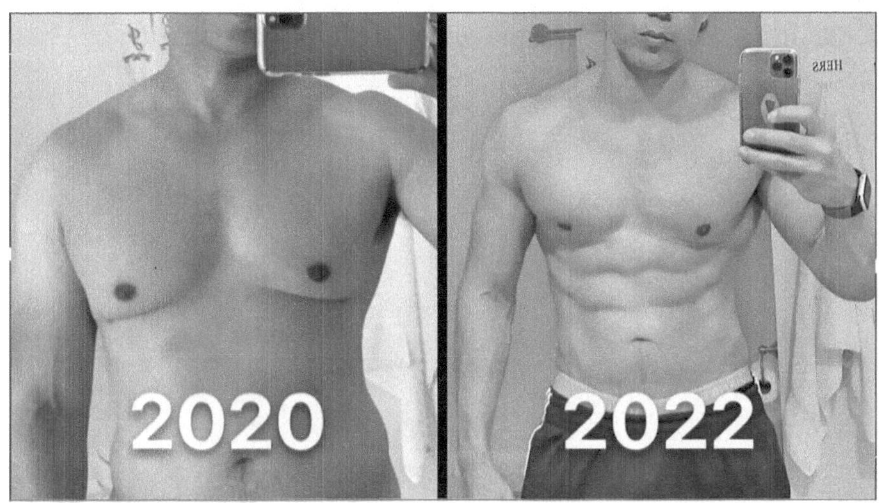

MY BODY TRANSFORMATION DUE TO MY HEALTH CONCERNS

Besides the health benefits, I started to see positive changes in the way I looked. I lost fat, gained muscle, and felt great. The morning routine became a part of my life that did not interfere with work or family. I had more energy and was better able to care for our disabled son. As I gained strength, I searched for new ways to challenge myself: I started training at a local martial arts gym to learn Brazilian jiu-jitsu (BJJ). BJJ is one of the most physically and mentally challenging activities to which I've ever dedicated myself. It is the greatest simulation for life-or-death combat without striking. The goal is to submit your training partner with various attacks that threaten injury to the extremities or strangulation. Yes, this sounds terrifying, but your safety in this form of training comes from the "tap-out." As soon as you feel that you are in a compromised position, you tap your partner or say "tap," and the attack stops. This style of training is amazing because it gives you the opportunity to train with individuals of various sizes, strengths, and levels of experience without undue fear of injury, provided you tap. You must learn to leave your ego at the door because failure to tap can lead to injury. One of the most remarkable lessons is that strength cannot compete with experience and mastery of technique.

In the beginning, the adrenaline surge can compromise your endurance, but as you become comfortable being in a compromised position, you learn how to protect yourself while remaining calm. During early training, from white belt to blue belt, learning the fundamentals is key. Even more important is the concept of learning how to survive and escape. Before attempting to submit your opponent with various techniques, you must gain a dominant position to control and pin your training partner so that a submission attempt is possible. This objective works both ways simultaneously, so it's like a physical game of chess. Among experienced belts, this process of dominating a training partner appears effortless. I have trained with black belts who control me so effectively that I feel like a kindergartner being held down by a high school linebacker. Most of these black belts are not stronger than I am, but their skill is so superior that strength doesn't matter. When I have competed against those who have more experience and greater strength, I might as well be an infant. This form of mastery is the closest thing to becoming Batman.

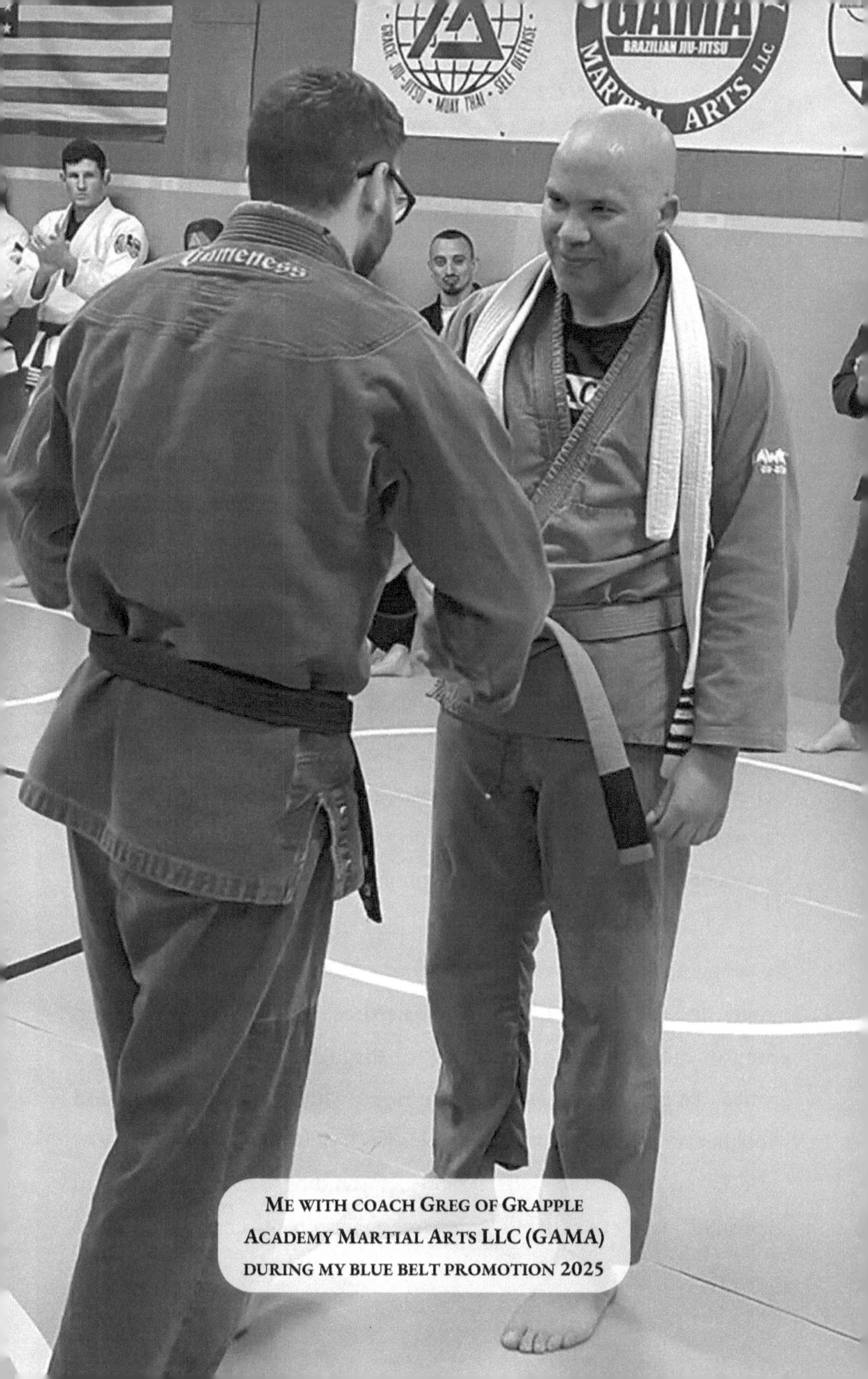

Me with coach Greg of Grapple Academy Martial Arts LLC (GAMA) during my blue belt promotion 2025

I've had a few minor injuries during my first year of training, but as I've gained experience and been promoted to blue belt, my respect for this remarkable martial art has grown significantly. I've also gained a great community of friends who share the same goals and fascination with this very humbling form of combat. As a surgeon, I am a somewhat unique participant in this activity, but once you put in the work and witness the skill others develop through training, it's hard to stop. The lessons learned from BJJ training can apply to other aspects of life. Becoming more attuned to your body's limits in various positions can help you avoid injuries in the operating room. In surgery, we spend long hours participating in physically demanding procedures. Some surgeons suffer neck and back injuries simply from poor posture. Some senior surgeons who spent decades performing long operations have developed a "surgeon's hunch," called kyphosis. I've always tried to maintain habits that protect me from such back problems, including adopting the best possible posture while operating. However, for large open cases, adjusting the bed height can only go so far in minimizing back strain. Despite these efforts, working deep in a patient's abdomen still presents ergonomic challenges.

Thankfully, technology has provided advantages that have aided in prolonging the careers of some surgeons who may otherwise have had to retire due to neck and back issues. Laparoscopic surgery has allowed surgeons to perform many operations through small incisions using a video camera and specialized instruments while standing upright and looking at a video monitor. While this has its advantages, long cases can still be taxing on the body because of standing the entire time and constantly using their hands. The game changer has been the addition of robotic surgery. Robotic surgery has evolved significantly over the years and is quickly becoming one of the favored approaches for laparoscopic surgery. The robot is connected to the patient through specialized adaptors placed by the surgeon. The robotic instruments are then controlled by the surgeon through an ergonomically adjusted console where the surgeon sits and views the surgical field. This console provides 3D optics for visualization inside the patient that is far superior to any flat-screen monitor. The hand controllers are capable of greater articulation than the human wrist, and the robot compensates for any small tremor that the surgeon may have. Most surgical disciplines have found a niche for this technology, and it continues to evolve. After a long day of performing cases robotically, the common neck and back discomfort often experienced after open and classic laparoscopic surgery is significantly reduced. The professional longevity of a surgeon can now be extended, and many are no longer forced into early retirement due to physical limitations associated with aging. Transitioning to robotic surgery is, in many ways, similar to becoming a surgical black belt, in that it allows surgeons to use their experience to deliver excellent surgery while minimizing injury to themselves.

CHAPTER 24

The End of My Story?

My commute home usually takes about 45 minutes without much traffic, and this was one of those days. I had just finished my third outpatient surgery of the day and was enjoying some music on my drive. I had this song stuck in my head called "I've Got to Live," by Sam Fischer, an omen for what was about to happen, perhaps. Without warning, I started to feel weak. There was no dizziness, no chest pain, but there was a feeling of something being wrong in my chest. I checked my Apple Watch and used the ECG feature to see if my heart rhythm was normal, and it was not. The tracing looked strange, and the watch could not say what was wrong, except that it detected an abnormality. I was not far from home and blamed the movement in the car for the reading being off. I thought there was no way I could have something wrong with me. I did weight training six days a week, went to jiu-jitsu classes two to three times per week, and even competed at local tournaments. I arrived home and sat down in the dining room to recheck the Apple Watch; I remained in the same abnormal rhythm. My wife checked my blood pressure and my pulse. There was no problem there, but the feeling that something was wrong in my chest persisted, so I went to the ER.

Heart concerns are a high priority, so when I shared what had happened with the triage nurse in the ER, I was quickly moved to a room, had labs drawn, and an ECG was performed. The ER doctor picked up the ECG, and a look of concern came over his face as he reviewed the tracing. Without delay, he said, "We are going to call cardiology; you are currently in a rhythm that is most often seen after someone has had a heart attack." I was speechless and scared. I said, "Okay," so as not to delay his call to the cardiologist with any questions.

My wife had been parking the car and had just walked in to join me. I briefed her on what was happening, and her eyes revealed her concern. As her questions about alternative explanations began, I was taken to another room, where I was met by the cardiologist, who performed an echocardiogram. He quickly introduced himself in a calm and professional tone but also shared that he wanted to get straight to work by performing the test to evaluate my heart function. He applied the cold gel to my chest, and it reminded me of my wife's ultrasounds when she was pregnant with our kids. As that thought crossed my mind, my oldest son, Tre, arrived. "Dad, are you okay?" Tre asked with growing concern. I often downplay my concerns, but I responded honestly. "I'm not sure." I looked to the cardiologist as he moved the ultrasound probe from one angle to the next and pushed buttons on the machine. I could not see the images, but his look of concern was enough to make me very uneasy. I asked him whether everything was okay, and he hesitated for a couple of seconds as he gathered his words, took a deep breath, and said, "Your heart function is not normal. You may have had a heart attack, so we are going to have you undergo an emergency angiogram." An angiogram is a procedure done with catheters to diagnose and treat areas of poor blood flow to the heart.

I immediately accepted what needed to be done but also felt panic about what would happen to my family if I were to die. I quickly began reminding my wife about the different life insurance accounts and the password to my laptop so that there would be no problem getting access to anything. After confirming that my wife had all the details she needed, a feeling of calm settled over me, and the fear went away. I had not accepted that I was about to die, but I knew that death was a possibility, and if it were to come, everything was going to be all right. I gave my life to Jesus many years ago, so I have faith that there is much more after this life comes to an end. I accepted that if it were my time to go, that would be alright. I had accomplished many things in life, had a wonderful family, a career that I loved and was good at, and had traveled the world, but all these things would mean nothing if I had not become right with the Lord. I had more that I wanted to do with my life to serve God beyond what I had already done. At this moment, I started to think about all the opportunities I could have taken to do more to help others, and I decided to commit to becoming a better representation of my Lord and Savior. If I were to live, I would do better.

Within minutes, I was rolled back to the procedure room, where they shaved the groin area and applied a cold, sterile prep solution before placing the sterile drapes. I was at Johns Hopkins, so our Chair of Surgery, Dr. Andrew Cameron (son of Dr. John Cameron, former Chair of Surgery at Hopkins), was kind enough to stop by and lend his support as I lay on the OR table with a sterile towel across my groin. I also had several of our residents working behind the scenes to help ensure all the pieces were falling into place, and there was direct communication with my former program director, Dr. Lipsett, who had always been a strong advocate for me. I was expecting to be completely under anesthesia for the procedure, but I was awake for the entire thing. The sharp stick of the needle in my groin to access the artery, followed by the burn of the local anesthesia, wasn't too bad. The pressure of the catheter being inserted was hardly noticeable. I felt some warmth as they injected the contrast to highlight the arteries supplying my heart. I listened to what was being said and was relieved to hear that there were no blockages. They did notice that my heart remained in the abnormal rhythm, for which they had no clear explanation.

I was admitted after the procedure for monitoring and for a trial of various medications to see if they could correct the abnormal heart rhythm. I could tell that something was still abnormal because I felt what I described as an empty feeling in my chest, like the Grinch; perhaps my heart was two sizes too small. The cardiologists found a medication that worked, but it was one that also carried the risk of causing life-threatening arrhythmias. I was relieved that they were able to break me out of this abnormal rhythm but concerned about the long-term effects. I was discharged on the new medication with a plan for further diagnostic testing to determine the etiology, or cause, of the problem.

They repeated the echocardiogram before discharge to ensure that my heart was functioning normally, and thank God it was. I could tell because that "empty" feeling had gone away.

I remained on the heart medication for several months while they conducted an extensive workup that included genetic testing, a cardiac MRI, multiple ECGs, and finally another invasive procedure with a cardiologist who specialized in heart arrhythmias. The plan for that procedure involved going to sleep this time while they accessed the groin vessels and then advanced into my heart to stimulate various regions from the inside to elicit the original arrhythmia again. If they could identify the area that was causing the arrhythmia, they could freeze those regions of the heart responsible for the abnormality to destroy that part of the tissue. Essentially, they would create a planned, focal heart attack. Again, I was not afraid, but again, I thought that if it were my time, I was ready. Before having the procedure, they had me stop the medication a few days in advance so that the arrhythmia would no longer be suppressed. Despite discontinuing the medication, I did not develop the strange sensation that I had previously experienced when the arrhythmia was present.

I still underwent the procedure. The plan was to stimulate all the regions within the heart while I was asleep so they could map out the areas that contracted normally and locate the region responsible for the abnormal rhythm. Sometimes, being under anesthesia can suppress the area responsible for the arrhythmia, so the plan was to awaken me in the middle of the procedure if they could not identify the problem area. They would then stimulate different parts of my heart again while I was awake to see whether this would trigger the abnormal rhythm that had originally been observed. Although I understood the plan, I hoped that it would not come to that. The idea of purposely being awakened during an invasive procedure with catheters in my heart and electrodes stimulating the tissue while I was awake was a bit much to handle. I knew too much and understood too much.

I was awakened by the voice of my cardiologist, who said, "We couldn't find the area that was causing the arrhythmia, so we are going to start mapping the area again, as we discussed, while you are awake." I acknowledged this with apprehension about what was about to happen. I imagined the little electrodes stimulating the inside of my heart, with my heart racing in response to the stimulation, and that is exactly what happened. I tried my best to remain silent as this was happening, but as my heart raced with a rapid flutter in my chest, I imagined the little needles poking all the way through my heart and causing a rupture that could lead to a life-threatening condition in which blood could leak from the heart. That scenario is incredibly rare, but because I knew it was possible, my mind went there. If that were to happen, the heart could collapse as blood leaked out and filled the space around the heart, which is enclosed within a thick layer of tissue that forms a protective sac called the pericardium. This condition is known as cardiac tamponade. If that were to occur, the heart would not be able to pump effectively, and I could die without emergency correction of this problem.

My heart raced, punctuated by very short, normal-feeling breaks. One episode seemed to last for a long stretch of time, and I asked, "Is that okay?" There was no answer. I repeated, "Hello? Is that normal? My heart is racing. Can you hear me?" Still no answer. I started to worry that

I was not actually speaking and that I had fallen into some dreamlike state, but then I heard my cardiologist say, "You're fine; we just have not seen any sign of that abnormal rhythm despite stimulating all the areas where we expected to find it." I felt some relief, but also some concern, because I wanted definitive treatment that could prevent the arrhythmia from returning. The procedure ended, and my cardiologist decided to follow up with me in a few weeks after having me wear a heart monitor to rule out any further episodes of arrhythmia while off the medications.

The heart monitor never detected the arrhythmia, and I never again felt any symptoms concerning its return. At my follow-up visit, I was cleared to return to all activities without restriction. The etiology of the arrhythmia was never clearly determined, but the outcome had a positive impact on my spiritual health and well-being. Nothing compares to the reality of facing death to make you reevaluate what is important in life. Although I had already given my life to Christ, I was not fully committing my life to serving others outside of what I did professionally as a surgeon. Again, I thought *I could have been doing more.* For years, I had been saying that I would begin doing more consistent outreach to people in need, but my busy schedule frequently became the reason I never found the time. I had turned down opportunities to focus on some of my interests in serving through global health initiatives in areas of need and had not returned to such efforts since my time as a resident in Rwanda. I had also fallen away from reading the Bible as consistently as I once did because I believed I did not have the time.

Facing the possibility of death and thinking about what I would say to Jesus when I met Him caused me to reflect deeply. I knew that I could have worked harder to serve Him through service to others. Jesus showed the way by how He lived, and I was not living to my full potential. I was not fully doing God's will. I was making excuses to remain comfortable and complacent. I had to make a difference so that when my time comes, I will not be afraid to see Jesus. I now begin each day with prayer and reading God's word. I look for opportunities to serve God by serving others, not only in my career, but also in my everyday life. I do not look forward to death, but I am no longer afraid of when that day comes. I am so thankful for the mysterious illness and suffering that changed me for the better and brought me closer to God. I pray that others can learn from my story and not have to face such trials in order to learn the lessons that I did.

CHAPTER 25

Hope for the Future

The world suddenly looked different. After my time in the hospital and a close encounter with the idea of leaving this world long before my expected time, the way I saw everything changed. For several years during my time as a surgical attending, I had plans to return to Africa to lend support to people in need, but because of the challenges of maintaining a busy practice and meeting obligations to my family, it was hard to find the time. The trip that I had been turning down for years because of my busy schedule was long overdue. My heart condition had miraculously resolved, so I had no excuse; I was committed to making the time to go. Dr. Zach Enumah had just completed his residency at Johns Hopkins, so this would be his first time going as a fully trained general surgeon. Zach had been making the trip each year with his father, Dr. Festus Enumah, who is also a surgeon and an author. They had identified a region with a large refugee camp that held more than 100,000 people from surrounding countries such as the Democratic Republic of the Congo and Burundi who had escaped war and persecution. The camp has served as a place for displaced people to live, but because of limited resources, there has been a great need for outside assistance to provide basic necessities such as fresh water, food, and medical care.

I was aware of the need for surgeons to help, but awareness through word of mouth does not come close to what is understood through firsthand experience. Being in the environment and seeing individuals in need with your own eyes does not allow for the rapid emotional disconnect that one may experience when watching a commercial or scrolling on social media about people suffering from starvation. When you encounter someone who is suffering and you possess the means to help, there is no changing the channel or turning away to ignore the sadness until a new advertisement about fast food captures your attention. Once one has made the decision to commit to helping people in need, the mind often returns to those left behind and to the question of when one can return to do more. That happened to me. The amazing efforts of healthcare professionals who dedicate their lives to people who have nothing to give beyond their gratitude exemplify some of the most remarkable people in the world. They do not do the work for money or praise, but because they feel it is their purpose to serve those in need. I am very fortunate to help people for a living through my skill set as a surgeon, but this does not come close to what many in the global health community are doing. I am paid to provide health care. To have a profession that allows me to help people and, at the same time, earn a wage to provide for my family is amazing, but I would be ashamed to pretend that what I do as a profession every day compares to the selflessness that so many have shown toward people like those trapped in the refugee camp I visited in Tanzania.

It took about a day of travel to reach the refugee camp located on the western side of Tanzania. This trip was quite special because we had a group of our Hopkins residents, along with residents and faculty from other institutions. Zach was already at the camp several days ahead of me with his father and his brother Sam, who is also a surgeon. The team had been working day and night in the camp, performing operations on people who had been waiting for several months to receive surgical care. I arrived toward evening and hit the ground running by joining in the last operation of the day. Each day, the group would round on all the patients from the previous day, along with those who remained on the ward, and then begin operating on patients who had been identified as having a surgical need, in order of urgency. We had a break room where we would grab a snack between cases but waited to eat together as a group at the end of the day at a restaurant just outside the refugee camp. Each day, we repeated the same routine and extended our hours into the night to address the long list of patients on the waiting list. Despite the long hours, the time passed quickly, and the work was incredibly rewarding. The people were very grateful, and despite their extremely difficult living conditions and limited resources, they still showed joy and peace in fellowship with one another. Some children had lost their parents due to war or illness, but individuals in the camp took them in and cared for them as their own. These individuals often had little more than a change of clothes as their possessions, yet they still sacrificed to help others.

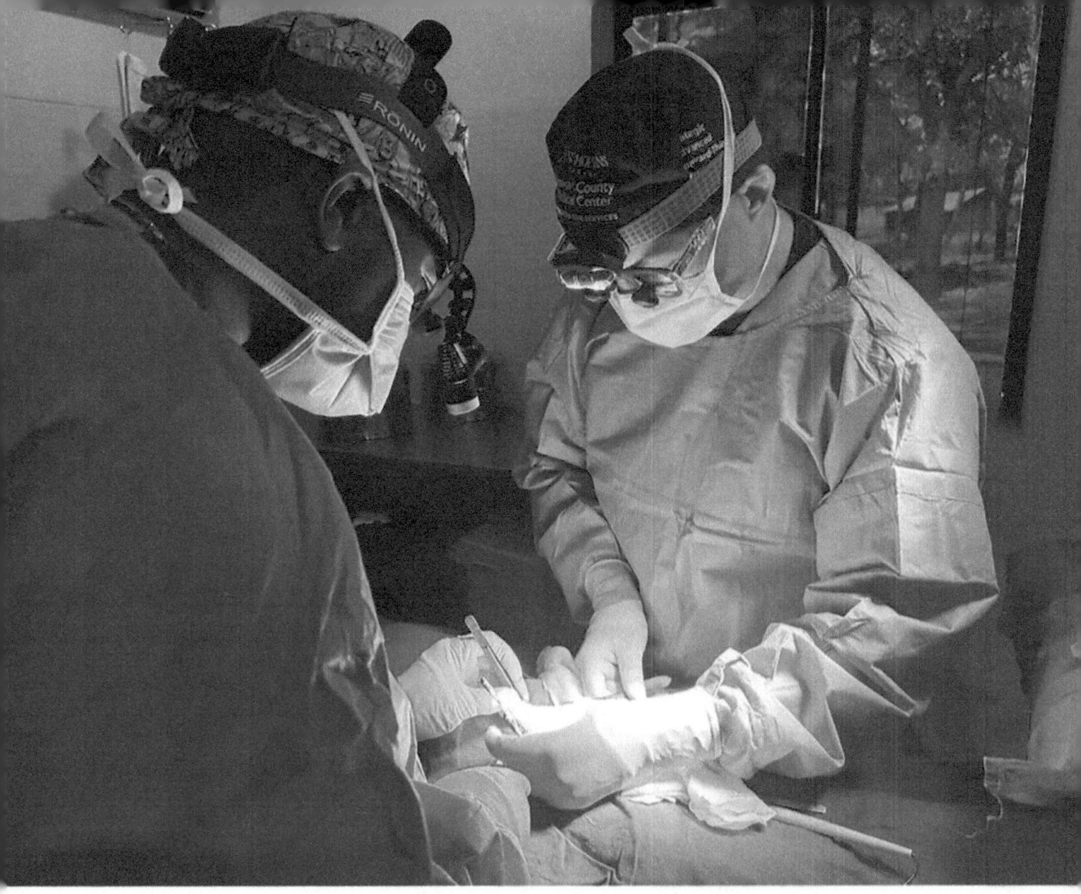

ME OPERATING WITH HOPKINS SURGICAL RESIDENT, DR. BROWN, ON AN INFANT IN THE REFUGEE CAMP IN TANZANIA, 2025

The love and joy that I saw among the refugees was inspiring. How can I complain about trivial things when they can still smile despite their extreme circumstances?

The trip to the refugee camp was transformative. Living and working in the United States is quite a privilege that many of us do not fully appreciate until we see what others are experiencing in other parts of the world. The challenges we face do not seem so overwhelming when compared to the conditions faced by people who must worry about finding clean water, food, shelter, and safety. Once you see, or, better yet, experience what it is like to lack the most basic human needs, it becomes difficult to feel discouraged about something as mundane as being stuck in traffic for an hour or not having the type of coffee that I usually order. This contrast in how we live compared to the people in the refugee camp softened my heart and changed the way I look at the world. The experience helped me appreciate what I have and inspired me to look for more opportunities to help others beyond what I do as a surgeon.

The following Christmas, my family decided to no longer spend thousands of dollars on gifts for each other. Instead, we chose to dedicate time and financial resources to helping others in need. Our previous focus on obtaining material possessions held no lasting value; such things push us away from God. By giving to others who are in need, our hearts can grow, and we store treasures in Heaven. It is truly better to give than to receive, and by serving others with our resources and talents, we strive to be more like Jesus, who lived as a man and gave His very life so that we may live. I think of the example that Jesus set, not only in sacrificing His life, but also in taking the humble role of washing the feet of His disciples as a way of teaching us that we should serve others.

A quote by Vivian Greene says, "Life isn't about waiting for the storm to pass . . . It's about learning to dance in the rain." Many people will face difficult situations in their lives, and the circumstances may at times be temporary, but what if they aren't? What if the challenge you are facing, this storm, is now the new normal in your life, like it is for Marcus and our family? You can spend a considerable amount of time and energy worrying about things you cannot change. A more productive way of handling difficult situations is to work around the challenges you face to find happiness and satisfaction. Turning to prayer is important, but even this can be done in a way that leads to disappointment when we don't get what we want. We often turn to God to ask for our will to be done, rather than asking to learn to accept His will. For as long as I can remember, I have prayed at the start of every day. Until recently, I spent the majority of this prayer time thanking God for the blessings I have been given and asking for things that I wanted: safety for my family, healing for those who are sick, guidance for difficult decisions, and so on. My prayer time was mostly one-sided, with very little time spent clearing my mind to give God the opportunity to speak to me. I have never heard an audible voice from God, either externally or in my head, but by clearing my mind and getting rid of all the background noise in the moment, I have experienced inspiration and guidance come to me in such a way that I believe it comes from God.

Sometimes we have so many things on our minds that we become distracted and unable to focus clearly on anything, let alone a potential power that cannot be seen. Many people experience some of their best ideas while in the shower. Some would argue that even this is a form of meditation where, instead of clearing your mind by focusing on your breath, you are focusing on the routine act of showering. The act of clearing my mind has been helpful to me, not only with patients in the clinic and in the operating room, but also in my interactions with friends and family. This is something that I still continue to work on so that I can give the best of myself to those I am with. With practice, learning to clear my mind of all distractions has given me a whole new perspective on life and how we should spend our time with each other. A true connection cannot easily be made while holding a conversation with your spouse if one eye is on the television and the other is on your smartphone. I have tried and failed many times.

Recognizing the importance of *quality* time when time is limited makes it easier to accomplish more without burning out emotionally. Physician burnout is a serious problem, and when we are not recognized as human beings with real feelings and emotions like everyone else, we can begin to behave like robots. We are already under high-stress circumstances when caring for patients and facing pressure to become more efficient with fewer resources. Many physicians work longer hours and see more patients, often with little time to eat or even go to the bathroom when needed. Once we begin to feel like robots, we start to lose empathy. We should always approach every patient encounter with the respect that we would expect for ourselves or a loved one. Unfortunately, as we become dehumanized as physicians, we can fall victim to the same emotional detachment toward our patients.

Over the years, I have learned to take time for myself as a way to avoid burnout. For me, this time is usually in the morning with prayer and meditation, followed by working on personal goals. Starting off my day focusing on personal growth allows me to feel accomplished and gives me the energy I need to focus on taking care of others. At the end of the day, before going to sleep, I reflect on the good things that happened and give thanks to God for them. Even when I have had a difficult day, I still think about the good things that are present in my life so that I do not lose sight of what is important. Despite some of the painful things that have happened in my life, I know that circumstances could always be worse. Giving extra attention or focus to negative experiences for the purpose of wallowing in my sorrows will only bring more negativity my way. After focusing on the good things in my life, I think briefly about my plan for the next morning, and then it's lights out.

My story is unique, but I am not alone. Others have experienced similar challenges throughout life and managed to keep going—as I have. I would like to think that my story can help those who have failed in some of the many ways that I have. It is possible to come from a broken home surrounded by poverty, drugs, and gang violence and then go on to break that cycle to create an environment free from those influences. It is possible to become a teenage parent and learn how to build a successful family. It is possible to have been forced out of regular high school due to failing grades, and to work hard enough to graduate and go on to college. It is possible to work 40 to 60 hours a week while attending college to support your family and still work toward your academic goals. It is possible to fail an entire semester in college, receive a below-average score on the MCAT, and still gain admission to the medical school of your dreams. It is possible to come from a weak academic background to then work hard and thrive in medical school, achieving performance in the 99th percentile on the medical board exam. It is possible for a kid from the ghetto to become a surgeon trained at one of the top surgical residency programs in the world. It is possible to raise and support a family on a surgical resident's income, even if barely. It is possible to survive the near death of a child. It is possible to learn how to adapt to the difficulties of caring for that child who was about to go off to college but, after a traumatic brain injury, has become blind, paralyzed on one side of the body, and has the cognitive ability of a four-to-five-year-old. It is possible to maintain hope for the future. It is possible to find happiness even before the storm passes. It is possible to learn how to dance in the rain.

Acknowledgments

I would like to give thanks first to my Lord and Savior, Jesus Christ, for I am lost without His grace and mercy. I was blessed with an amazing, beautiful, and courageous wife, Rosina. Rosina is the love of my life, and with the help of the Lord working in both of us, she has helped shape me into the man I am today. We have grown up together and formed a bond through our love that has withstood the tests of time, tragedy, poverty, and devastation. To my son, Tre, you were the first reason for me to change for the better. I am so proud of the hardworking man you have become. You have followed your passion as a writer and inspired me to want to write beyond these pages. To my son, Marcus, I know in my heart that the tragedy that you went through was allowed to happen for a reason. You have taught me to be more appreciative of life by witnessing your pure joy that you exude every day. You are a blessing to the world, and I know that someday your body will be restored to its intended glory. To my daughter, Danielle, you will always be my baby girl. I am so proud of you. You have become an amazing, thoughtful, caring, intelligent, and independent woman. To my fellow faculty members and residents at Hopkins, you are all the reason I have stayed with the institution and never left. The residents are the future of surgery, and it is an honor and privilege to have a role in their training. At one of the most difficult times in my life, the Hopkins family was there for my family when we had no other support.

I want to thank all the beta readers who helped me by following my chapter releases through my website, along with my son, Tre, for the first round of edits. My wife read every chapter and provided support for the accuracy of our life's history, which was shared in this memoir. I also want to thank Robin Schroffel of Golden Starling Publishing and Dina Ruiz Eastwood for the last round of copyediting (Dina became a friend through social media and volunteered her valuable time without fee). Finally, I am grateful for all of the friends, family, and social media supporters who have offered so much love and support throughout this process.

About the Author

D r. James Harris Jr. is a general surgeon at Johns Hopkins Howard County Medical Center, where he serves as the Chair of Surgery and holds an academic position as Associate Professor in the School of Medicine and Associate Program Director for the Johns Hopkins Surgical Residency Program. He is married to his high school sweetheart, Rosina, and they have three adult children: Tre, who is married and works as a college English adjunct professor and aspiring writer; Marcus, who had a traumatic brain injury and has lived at home since his accident; and Danielle, who is engaged and works as a biologist. Dr. Harris' "Unusual Path to Becoming a Surgeon" began when he was a child of poverty, raised in a crack house during the crack epidemic in Fresno, California. His path looked more likely to lead to destruction, based on the troubles of his adolescence, the various crimes he participated in as a teenager, and becoming a father at fifteen. But through God's grace, there was an unexpected transformation. His story of resilience and determination led him to achieve all his dreams, but his early struggles were only preparing him for some of the most difficult challenges he would ever face. His story is one of survival, and it is meant to be shared with others who are going through impossible times and who feel there is no hope. This story is meant to prove that despite seemingly impossible odds, God has a purpose for your life, and you should never give up.